To Zuzana and Branko,

With thanks for all your lovely notes.

Memory

All alone in the moonlight

I can smile at the old days

I was beautiful then

I remember the time I knew what happiness

was

Let the memory live again

- **Tim Rice - From Andrew Lloyd Webbers musical "Cats"**

Introduction

When I was writing my first book in The Secret Healer Series *The Complete Guide to Clinical Aromatherapy and The Essential Oils of The Physical Body* twelve months ago, I woke one night very agitated that I had spoken about the Egyptians and their usage of plant medicine but had not cited evidence to support it. This concerned me and so I wrote to the eminent Egyptologist Prof. Joann Fletcher and asked her for help. Generously she was able to give me a large number of places to research as well as contact details for Dr. Lise Manniche, the Egyptologist responsible for the beautiful book *Sacred luxuries*: *fragrance, aromatherapy, and cosmetics in Ancient Egypt*. We each spoke at length about how we thought they may have come to know the properties of the plants and agreed that the physicians of old had **hypothesized, experimented and watched.**

Today, we have the benefits of a great deal of their knowledge gathered through archaeological finds of papyri. We have Galen's second century discovery that disease has a prognosis and that illness may come from internal or external factors, rather than being due to some wrath from the gods. We have endless tomes of herbal medicine and we have laboratory evidence for *some* of the things that plant medicine can do.

But we are merely a snapshot on a scientific timeline. We look at the past, sitting in the present, wondering at the medicine of the future.

We have a great deal of proof for the efficacy of our medicine now, but there is still a mammoth amount of data to find. This book takes the evidence we have about Clary Sage and says *what if....*

Many authorities describe Clary Sage as having an oestrogen-like structure and thus suggest that it mimics oestrogen in the bloodstream. But, as yet, however there is no strong scientific evidence to support this. (There is none to discredit the claim either, it is important to state). So, we wonder, what if *it does*?

You think you know oestrogen?

Yep, I did too.

I don't think I am boasting when I say my endocrinology knowledge is good, and yet I was shaken to the core to read of all the new discoveries into what doctors now understand that oestrogen can do, how it affects our health and the terrifying implications into disease when its levels begin to drop. That applies to men and women, incidentally.

In this book, rather than walking around laboratories checking that our rats and mice are OK after their various stress tests, we wear the mantles of the great physicians and philosophers of the past. We sit amongst Dioscorides, Theophastrus and Pliny and discuss their findings about the plant with the new clinical findings about female sex hormones. We ask if the last ten years research into oestrogen affect what we know about Clary Sage medicine and if it is ever categorically proven to be estrogenic, how many more people could it help?

Well, without spoiling the next 120 or so pages, we are not only talking about menstruation and menopause, it is now known that oestrogen affects heart disease, respiratory dysfunction, cognition, mood, skeletal problems. In, fact it is now known that it has at least 400 functions in the body. That it protects the brain and when oestrogen declines so does general and mental health.

Now there, is of course, hormone replacement therapy, and more specifically *oestrogen* replacement therapy, which is made from the urine of pregnant mares...but what if we could protect ourselves from these diseases through the essential oil of a plant? What if we could guard against Alzheimer's disease, heart problems and stroke? What if we could hold onto those last few memories, when we are sat in the old people's home, for just a few weeks longer?

If you learn nothing about Clary Sage from this, and I hope that you do, I feel sure you will learn an extraordinary amount about hormones and neurology in particular. Most of all, I hope to give every woman an insight into just how spectacular her body is and to show that the Mind Body Spirit is *quintessentially* glued together by oestrogen.

Finally, when that glue begins to deteriorate, to show how that strangely nutty scented oil, that many of us thought of as a simply a gentler version of common sage, might just be the most flexible healing medicine of them all. The question is though...how on earth does one go about using it?

Learn when to use and when *not* to use Clary Sage in

- Poly Cystic Ovarian Syndrome
- Period Pains
- Perimenopause
- Menopause
- Breathing Problems
- Wounds
- Anxiety
- Insomnia
- Depression

Understand hormones from the inside out and then benefit from 50 recipes of how to use Clary Sage.

Can you smell the lovely nutty fragrance drifting on the wind changing the face of female medicine? Come with me. Let's walk through her fields, drawing our fingers through the flowers, and find out the truth about "nature's own estrogen" and how we can use it to improve menopause, menstruation problems, inflammatory problems such as osteoarthritis and restless legs.

Table of Contents

Before we begin...

At 4am Sept 27th I was awakened by the brightness illuminating my bedroom. The supermoon forbade me to sleep. So I went downstairs to get a drink and checked my facebook as the kettle boiled.

This book originates from a facebook post I was tagged in that night. Later that evening the Earth was plunged into darkness in a lunar eclipse and I started to wonder about the strange co-incidence I had found earlier in the day, that the oil occupying my thoughts was ruled by the moon and that all of her medicine seemed to be hormonal (menstruation, menopause both come from the word stem pertaining to the cycles of the moon.)

I was asked, in the post, if Clary Sage would be a good choice to make a soap for a friend who was struggling to become pregnant. She had read that it could help infertility. I immediately recalled that according to many sources Clary Sage exhibited oestrogen-like traits so at a glance it might be useful and yet....As the medical history of the friend became clear, I realised that hundreds, if not thousands of women may be making their fertility issues worse by using this wrongly chosen oil.

I pondered on that...

Then as always seems to happen, I received a message from Aromatika.hu to ask me if I could write something on Clary Sage. I am beginning to think that Gergely Hollodi might be my writing's guardian angel! I had already researched a great deal on Menopause earlier in the autumn for NAHA and it seemed jigsaw pieces might be collecting again.

So the book grew and grew. My desk got messier and my head ached more and more. But the research got ever more fascinating, so I searched, read and read compulsively. And oestrogen became my newest obsession.

Which brings me to my point and to a wry apology...

When I was 9, I had the most dreadful teacher Miss Baker. She looked, for all the world, like The She Devil but with more facial hair and she was goddamn horrible to me about spellings. Mainly, because I wouldn't learn them. Then one week she threatened me with...I can't even remember what but it worked and I learned them. I got 20/20 and was expecting praise but instead the vile cow made me stand on my chair and said "You make me want to be sick in the corner." Which was pleasant, I thought. Anyway, in that test was the word oestrogen. It seemed to me that I had learned the wretched word for no good reason. But it appears not...so I am really not going to change it to US spelling I am afraid, even though I will confess that most of the research I have found comes with an E at the beginning of the word. The nine year old me would never forgive me. So, brace yourself Americans, you are going to flinch about...100 times. Sorry!

So without anymore ado...let's start thinking about this oil, Clary Sage.

The Chemistry of Clary Sage

As you all know, the chemistry of an oil often leaves me cold. I understand its construction and what each of the constituents might mean to the properties of that oil, but for me it is the ancient wisdoms and new neuroscientific discoveries that light my fire.

Not so with Clary Sage. I suppose mainly because there is so much disagreement about what it can and can't do, mostly in terms of pregnancy. The chemistry of Clary Sage is fascinating, not least because it shows just how small a component of one chemical can be and still make the most extraordinary changes to the body.

Chemistry is the reason why we are told to steer clear of Clary Sage's sister, Common Sage in most cases. In her chemistry, thujone is problematic and if you even look at the anatomy of the plant, our *Salvia sclarea* has a strong robust stem, where *officinalis* has tiny hairs demanding you treat it gently. *Salvia sclarea* is easier to handle.

Interestingly Clary Sage has the highest number of esters of any essential oil I can think of. Can you remember making esters at school in chemistry? They smelled like pear drops. Esters are lovely gentle components. They combine an acid and an alcohol, so each cancels the other's harshness out. It is a wonderfully neutral oil.

Medicinally, the properties of esters in an oil are:

- sedative

- antispasmodic
- antifungal
- anti- microbial

So, if you wanted be lazy and only wanted learn the properties of the oil through this chemistry, you could surmise that since CS comprises of just over 70% esters (depending in where it was grown) this would be a good indication of what the oil can do.

And you would be right.

Esters appear in essential oils a lot, because they give plants their delicious herby/fruity notes. As a plant ripens and matures, the esters increase and so we get a sweeter more rounded fragrance. You might remember from my Complete Guide that linalool, over time, will mature into linalyl acetate. One of the highest concentrations of esters in CS is linalyl acetate (comprising about 55% of the complete oil). Next in concentration is linalool.

Linalool

This constitutes about 15% of Clary Sage oil. So again, this is a precursor to linalyl acetate.

Now, linalool, we have met before because she played a starring role in the research in the Sweet Basil book. Scientists now agree that it is of fundamental importance in the fight against both depression and also inflammation. Incidentally, because of the repetition between the books, I have chosen not include research into linalool in this book, however reading those papers in the Sweet Basil book will only serve to improve your understanding of the far reaching potential of Clary Sage as a therapeutic agent, though that specific constituent.

Sclareol

In Clary Sage essential oil, sclareol usually constitutes just under 2% of the oil (although it can be as high as 7% depending on where it comes from). Sclareol is a solid component and has a very low volatility which makes it very hard to gauge on a gas chromatography reading. In the absolute, which is solid, it makes up a massive 70%. I guess that may mean that the E/o reading may not be completely reliable as to the true levels in the bottle! It is difficult, but not impossible to use the absolute in aromatherapy (You can still inhale it of course, although massage is not very easy). It is more often used in perfumery and as you can imagine is rich, and mouth-wateringly luxurious. In aromatherapy, we use the essential oil.

In a 1990 study by French aromatherapists Franchomme and Penoel, stated that the beneficial effects of Clary Sage were related to this constituent *sclareol* which was almost identical in structure to human oestrogen.

As such, they say, Clary Sage exercises an oestrogen like quality....

But in complete opposition this, in a 2007 paper *Biological activity of diterpenoids isolated from Anatolian Lamiaceae plants* Gülaçtı Topçu and Ahmet C. Gören classified sclareol as a labdane derivative and according to Tisserand and Young this would mean that sclareol would have *no* such estrogenic properties at all. In his 2010 blog post "Is Clary Sage Estrogenic" Tisserand writes

"Both estradiol and butylparaben contain a phenol functional group: a hydroxyl group (OH) attached to a benzene ring. The phenolic structure is important for estrogenicity, as is the presence of a second ring (Anstead et al 1997, Blair et al 2000). However, sclareol does not contain a phenolic structure, it doesn't even contain a benzene ring. Sclareol is a labdane diterpene, and this class of molecule does not incorporate estrogen-like structures, nor is it noted for estrogenic activity (Topçu and Gören 2007).

Therefore, on the basis of its structure, sclareol is unlikely to have any estrogenic action. Even if sclareol was estrogenic, at about 4% of Clary Sage oil, it would have to have a very high binding affinity for estrogen receptor sites for the essential oil to have any effect, and this is extremely unlikely."

He then goes on to say:

And, I'm not saying that sclareol could not possibly be estrogen-like, I'm just saying there's no evidence that it is, nor does its structure suggest such an effect.

And, to balance the argument he points out that a component of sclareol known as **13 epi-sclareol** has been found to inhibit breast and uterine cancers, in vitro, seemingly through **some kind of interaction with estrogen receptors.**

In *The Science of Essential Oils*, Kurt Schnaubelt tells us *"Through its sclareol content, Clary Sage has an estrogen-like quality and is used to ease premenstrual syndrome."*

Jane Buckle explains in *Clinical Aromatherapy in Nursing* "Essential oils such as rose, cypress or Clary Sage can be helpful when used in a hydrosol spray or spritzer sprayed around the face, neck, and shoulders during a hot flash. A few drops of peppermint added to the mix is wonderfully cooling. Essential oils that could be used for estrogen support include fennel, sage and aniseed. Geranium and rose give added support."

And whilst it might be easy to think that Clary Sage needs to be ingested or at least massaged into the system in *Toxicity Myths: the Actual Risks of Essential Oil Use, Ron Guba* asserts that something different might be happening.

"Other essential oils that have suggested menstrual-regulating effects,

through a long history of traditional use and/or significant results in clinical experience include: Clary Sage, Sage (Salvia officinalis), Lovage, Angelica Root, Niaouli and Cypress. In all such cases, the effects appear due to a secondary effect via the anterior pituitary, not by the addition of "hormone-like" compounds. The reported effects of the essential oil of Clary Sage (Salvia sclarea) bear this out. Many anecdotal reports have been given to the effects on menstruation by only inhalation of the essential oil."

Interesting.....

So, on one hand experts tell us that the Clary Sage changes hormones, but then several industry authorities dispute that and one in particular says...erm no...it is not the actual oil that changes the hormone, it's that it affects the pituitary which in term affects *secretion* of the hormones it produces, which consequently then, in turn, affects the oestrogenic levels.

So then...inhalation of the oil will be enough to bring about menstrual changes. And actually, of course, inhalation will be faster than rubbing it on, because the olfactory pathway is an autobahn into the bodymind.

Oestrogen, Sm'oestrostrogen!

Do we care how it happens?

Nah, not really at this point, personally I just care that it *in* practice it certainly *seems to*.

In truth, we still don't know *how* sclareol affects oestrogen, because no-one has been able to give us categorical proof yet.

Is your head ready to explode...?

Yep mine too. And apologies now...because it only gets worse! (Or better if you are an aromatherapist who wants to make someone better just by an essential oil, of course!)

Let's have a break from science for a bit and take a trip through Clary Sage history.

The History of Clary Sage

Historical references to Clary Sage are found in notations about a plant called Horminum, or Orminum. I am grateful to Tess Anne Osbaldeston for her meticulous translation of Dioscorides *De Materia Medica* for insights into this. Previously, I had found many references to Dioscorides, Pliny and Theophastrus citing the plant but scoured all of their works with no success. I was beginning to wonder if we were labouring under some kind of strange delusion (That would not be outside of the realms of possibility for a plant ruled by the moon after all!) Eventually a little door opened a crack with the ancient name...and I was in!

So in ancient texts it is listed as *Horminum pyrenaicum*, sometimes Clary and sometimes Gallitricum.

Where normally I might be able to go 5,000 years, the European record keeping is not as good as it was in Ancient Egypt for example, and predominately, it is a European plant, and is thought to originate from Syria. So, we have some Roman writings, then as ever a break in recording during The Dark Ages as Europe went into cultural decline and we have to wait until after the renaissance when Tudor sources, and later, give us a helping hand with evidence. In any case, it has been very difficult to find ancient information on this plant.

Dioscorides tells us...

Cultivated horminum is an herb similar to marrubium [you and I would know this as horehound] *in the leaves, but the stalk is four-cornered and half a foot high. There are abnormal growths similar to husks around this (as it were) looking towards the root, in which are two different types of seed. In the wild it is found round and dark, but in the other it is somewhat long and black. Use is made of this and it is also thought that a decoction (taken as a drink with wine) is an aphrodisiac. With honey it cleans away argema* [small white ulcer on the cornea], *and also white spots on the corneas of the eyes; and smeared on with water it dissolves oedema and extracts splinters. The herb (applied) does the same things. The wild one is stronger; as a result it is mixed with compound ointments (especially with gleucinum* [no translation known]*). The Romans call it geminalis, and the Dacians, hormia.* [Just in case you are interested the Dacians were an Indo-European people located around the Carpathian Mountains and Black Sea which we would now call Eastern Europe, Romania, Poland Hungary etc]

Many sources cite Clary Sage as being mentioned by Theophrastus, and it is, although in no more interesting statement in that he notices that it seems not to be eaten by cattle! He gives no further insights into use in either "Enquiry into Plants" or "Of Odours". This does tell us, though, that the plant was known to the Romans.

Pliny mentions it very briefly, in Historia Naturalis, as being a food that can change character when used in the diet. This seemingly innocuous comment makes me wonder about many things I have uncovered through the book.

How does it change character?

When I began the research, wine immediately sprang to mind. One of the reasons we say do not use large concentrations of CS in aromatherapy is because it *"stupefies"*, to use the word that was given in my own study notes. I couldn't quite picture what that would mean in practice. Then, I discovered that even today, in Germany, Clary Sage is called Muscatel Sage, because decoctions of Clary taste very much like the muscatel grape. But when it is added to wine, it makes you incredibly drunk in a very short time. Hence, it became standard practice to adulterate the wine with our plant. Then by the 16th Century this practice had been absorbed into English beer making too. This time they replaced the hop, which was far more expensive to produce. Potentially, no-one would be any the wiser whilst they were knocking back tankard after tankard, until they woke next morning with a chronic hangover. Too much Clary Sage...will give you a headache, with beer or without!

Now as the research has opened out...I think that it might have the capacity to change the character in a *different* way...and we will come back to that in a moment.

It was introduced to England in 1562, after having been native to Syria, Italy, Southern France and Switzerland. It was a useful and easy crop to grow because it will pretty much thrive in any soil that is not wet. (Often the roots will rot in English winters though, as the soil does not have chance to dry out.)

John Gerald, in fact describes several varieties of Clary Sage growing in England in his *Generall Historie of Plantes* (written 1597), each time referring to them as either Horminum or Gallitreum. He describes it as *"growing in diverse barren places in almost every country, especially in the fields of Holbourne neare to Grayes Inne and at the end of Chelsea"*. I love this imagery and that the thought that any plant might now prosper in what is now very much Millionaire's Row in the midst of a sprawling metropolis.

In 1710 William Salmon described a number of varieties of the *common clary. He speaks of Horminum commune, Horminum sativum var. dioscorides,* (or *the true clary of dioscorides*) Yellow Clary, *Callus jovis* and the small and garden clary, *Horminum humiles germanicum* also refered to as *Gallatricum alterum Geraldi.* The last species had been classified by John Gerald when he brought it over from the continent, evidently taking great pains to trace its origins right back to the Latin and Greek names in *his* herbal.

William Salmon is a fascinating source although is seldom quoted. Quite a rock star of his generation, a real live anarchist, he was all but forgotten after his death. His work *The English Herbal* is perhaps better remembered by the name *"Botonalgia"*. (There is a link to a scan of the manuscript in the bibliography. It is worth looking just for the illustrations.)

He was an outcast, really, not least because of British snobbery. He was Jamaican born and had been trained by someone who was not seen as a very good mentor. In fact, he was seen as a bit of a charlatan, which earned him the title "Mountebank" [one who tricks or deceives others for money].

Very little is known about his life but when I looked him up in the Oxford Dictionary of National Biography, Philip K. Wilson tells us: *"Contemporaries claimed that as a boy Salmon was apprenticed to a mountebank, whom he served as a 'wachum' or 'zany', and amused audiences by 'tumbling through a hoop' or with 'tricks of legerdemain and slight of hand'; he also 'made speeches and wrote Panygyricks in praise of his master's Panaceas. He wrote Almanacks to direct the taking of his medicines, and made the stars vouch for their virtue.'"*

This self proclaimed "Doctor of Physic" was extremely prolific and wrote treaties on everything from apothecary to the symbolisms of hand gestures, to surgery and figurative drawing. Remember too, the context of the time he was living in. The 18th century was a time of great knowledge growth, of exploration and fantastic new technology. The printing press was power and he used it to his full potential. He writes many books, but also it is very easy to find many adverts in newspapers of the period where he is claiming some testimonial to his herbal cures. He was clearly a very astute marketeer.

Possibly the finest of his "product placement" came about when he moved from his original place of consultation with his patients – in the local tavern – to a new premises smack opposite St Bartholomew's Hospital in London. Any "customers" the hospital turned away found their way to Salmon's establishment and he created a very nice little business, thank you very much.

He would prescribe his pills with some very suspect ingredients, cast astrological charts and even profess to perform alchemy…and he was very successful. But the scorn from the establishment continued.

I just thought I would write a bit about him because he was potentially the most successful physician of his time and he just seems to remind me of *someone* somehow. He worked hard. He was very good at his craft but his marketing was spectacular for his time. He was savvy but he never shook off that mantle of "Well, you know what his training was like…" and how often do you see that stated in a rather disparaging ways on social networks these days? Is it only me or can anyone else see parallels with a certain *Young* man and his essential oils too? Clever marketer, slightly dubious educational background, loved by many, hated and distrusted by a great number too…?

Anyway, despite the lengths he goes to with his classification he writes very little about usage of Clary Sage at the time, and so one could be forgiven for thinking none were really ascribed. But as ever our wonderful Nicholas Culpepper saved the day and I should point out that Culpepper precedes *Gary,* oops I mean William by almost a century, his herbal being written in 1634.

So what does our Nick have to say:

"CLARY - Or more properly clear-eye.

Description. Our ordinary garden clary hath four square stalks, with broad, rough, wrinkled, whitish, or hoary green leaves, somewhat evenly cut in on the edges, and of a strong sweet scent, growing some near the ground, and some by couples upon stalks. The flowers grow at certain distances, with two small leaves at the joints under them, somewhat like the flowers of sage, but smaller, and of a whitish blue colour. The seed is brownish, and somewhat flat, or not so round as the wild. The roots are blackish, and spread not far, and perish after the seed time. It is usually sown, for it seldom rises of its own sowing.

Place. This groweth in gardens.

Time. It flowereth in June and July, some a little later than others, and their seed is ripe in August, or thereabouts.

- *Government and virtues. It is under the dominion of the Moon. The seed put into the eyes clears them from motes, and such like things gotten within the lids to offend them, as also clears them from white and red spots on them.*

- *The mucilage of the seed made with water, and applied to tumours, or swellings, disperseth and taketh them away;*
- *as also draweth forth splinters, thorns, or other things gotten into the flesh.*
- *The leaves used with vinegar, either by itself, or with a little honey, doth help boils, felons, and the hot inflammations that are gathered by their pains, if applied before it be grown too great.*
- *The powder of the dried root put into the nose, provoketh sneezing, and thereby purgeth the head and brain of much rheum and corruption.*

The seed or leaves taken in wine, provoketh to venery.

- *It is of much use both for men and women that have weak backs, and helpeth to strengthen the reins: used either by itself, or with other herbs conducing to the same effect, and in tansies often.*
- *The fresh leaves dipped in a batter of flour, eggs, and a little milk, and fried in butter, and served to the table, is not unpleasant to any, but exceedingly profitable for those that are troubled with weak backs, and the effects thereof.*
- *The juice of the herb put into ale or beer, and drank, bringeth down women's courses, and expelleth the after-birth.*

I do like it when I find a plant that "provoketh to venery", I am considering writing a book about aphrodisiacs and calling it that! There is something so deliciously down and dirty about it isn't there somehow! Given that we also know that it is going to have you sozzled I would suggest this venery might also be the sort that one might have regretted in the morning. Tankards swigging, sawdust floors, buxom bosoms a-heaving…ah yes I can see it now. The good side of course, is if you did jump off the wardrobe and strain your back…clary can help that too!

So now he finishes with

"It is an usual course with many men, when they have gotten the running of the reins, or women the whites, they run to the bush of clary; maid, bring hither the frying-pan, fetch me some butter quickly, then for eating fried clary, just as hogs eat acorns; and this they think will cure their disease forsooth; whereas when they have devoured as much clary as will grow upon an acre of ground, their backs are as much the better as though they had pissed in their shoes; nay, perhaps much worse."

Confused dot com?

I was too. Now read it again, with the knowledge that "running of the reins" and "whites" in women, refers to the discharge of gonorrhea.

But does it work we all want to know?

He answers:

"We will grant that clary *strengthens* the back; *but* this we deny, that the *cause* of the running of the reins in men, or the whites in women, lies in the back, (though the back may sometimes be weakened by them) and therefore the medicine is as proper, as for me when my toe is sore, to lay a plaister on my nose."

So, he says "no gonorrhea patients, today" then. Oh well, can't say that I'm disappointed.

Going back to the original text we find that charmingly, gents would clear their noses with it around you (no matter how dashingly the light glints off your armour, I'll not be dropping my handkerchief for you, kind Sir) but more usefully we discover that we find he used it like a kind of drawing ointment, removing splinters and extruding boils. This echoes Dioscorides thoughts.

You will notice he calls it Clear Eye. Don't confuse it with EyeBright which is a different herb, but that "clear" is where its name clary comes from and actually Salvia sclaria means Salvia= to save Sclaria = clear.

Some of the texts from the Middle Ages also refer to it as Oculus Christi, or Eye of Christ, which perhaps pertains to the gentle salve for the eyes, or maybe its ability to help you perceive reason and insights more simply. I don't know. I couldn't find out. Either way, both would be true.

What I find far more interesting though is how similar the name Horminum is to the word hormone….

Ruling Planets

So as we sit in our 17th Century garden and contemplate the properties of the plant, we do not have the benefit of a petri dish or a centrifuge, all we have is the observations of the plant and some battered old books to fall on. We can look at the big droopy flowers languid and ripe with oil, and see that she is fertile. The broad strong stems tell us she is robust and hardy and since she is found in dry arid places, that she can be relied upon to cool in times of great heat.

What else?

We found out earlier that Culpepper details Clary Sage under moon ruler ship but I have also found a great many other sources also say under mercury. It is a strange dichotomy, but as the story unfolds it seems that *both* are indeed true. Let's begin by thinking about moon medicine.

See what you think.

Moon Medicine

In astrological study there is no distinction between male and female, so that means that we cannot say the sun is masculine and the moon is feminine. More correctly we *can* say that the moon communicates feminine principles and more pertinently feminine aspects of the psyche. In Jungian terms (as in Carl Jung's psychological hypotheses) we say that the moon represents the *anima*.

The anima and animus represent the entirety of feminine psychology. The *anima* is the **female qualities that a man possesses** and the *animus* is the **male qualities in a woman's make up**. Jung described how many of us turn our attention away from the fact that we have a genetic make up that carries markers of the opposite sex; they are part of us, yet many of us find it hard to embrace them.

The unconscious however, is always steered by the anima (or animus) and so often we will react unconsciously, not truly understanding why this has happened.

He wrote far more about the anima, the female aspect in a man, not least because he felt that men's sensitivities were more often suppressed to conform to societal stereotypes (remember we are talking about early Twentieth Century theories which do not have quite the same cultural significance today). He spoke of how the anima related to softness in the personality, nurturing and not least how a man felt about women, or indeed related to them.

The anima qualities are very much reflected in the context of moon energy. They are intuitive, nurturing and gentle. And whilst we cannot say they belong to women, they are most definitely ascribed to the feminine part of nature.

<u>**Moon energy is triggered, not activated.**</u> It is reflected in the way you feel about yourself before you even have the thought to ask yourself about it. It is deeply ingrained in your shadow and whilst some might say moon medicine is about the unconscious, I prefer to think of it as what we are unconscious *of…* In other words, we might have an unconscious reaction but it is that strange man holding a memory silently at gunpoint in the recesses of our mind that we are unconscious of. We have no awareness of why that particular memory sets off behaviour patterns we have, only perhaps that it does. And when the moon eventually breaks through the clouds, hopefully she will shine her medicine's light brightly enough bring him into light. Certainly this is the healing of moon ruled plants such as Clary Sage.

The key to understanding moon energy is to remember that she does not have her own power source. She is a luminary entirely dependent on the light of the sun. Her light is reflected and reflec*tion* is the medicine of her glow. She requires us to sit in peace, think and to reflect, and then she will allow us to hear her whispers.

I have to be honest and say that I am stunned by the strange coincidence that brought the lunatic fixation into my consciousness this time. It feels like the moon shook me awake that night to show me another molecule of emotion that I kept overlooking.

I suppose I was destined to fall prey to the lunar trap, Cancerian baby that I am. The moon represents our psychological character, and the endless unravelling of clues that seem to run everywhere and yet nowhere at once *is* entirely my cup of tea. The interesting thing about moon medicine of course, is just like her cycles there is a kind of fluctuating and changedness to the pattern and it is affected by external factors, I suppose. I am *always* drawn into chaotic research, it's like a magnetic charge to me, but my menstrual cycle will determine whether I giggle with frustration or throw the books out of the shed window!

The moon represents your very earliest learnings, those ancestral patterns passed down through your DNA and of course, that would also cover that which you have learned in utero about your mother's feelings for you. It is about nurturing and feelings of belonging. Moon medicine highlights the degree to which you have them and whether you are capable of them.

When the moon casts her glow it is likely we will gain an understanding as to how these parts of ourselves come to be a little awry. Most pertinently it is related to maternal instincts and understanding the needs of the infant. We might think of the rise of the anima as being a new dad who faces pink, wrinkly and smelly challenges he'd always deftly sidestepped before. Or we just as likely might find that the figure in the darkness who is pulling our internal strings is actually a very distressed child who has something to say. Clary Sage helps us to gently pull out a seat and listen as the tears flow and lets the aching soul choke out its perceived pains.

So the principles we associate with medicines and lessons from the moon are fundamentally mothering and nurturing. Feelings, and becoming more connected to one's emotions. Dependency and moodiness and we are looking to instil (or balance) a sense of openness and vulnerability.

I wonder, how do *you* experience the scent of Clary Sage? For as we know, everyone of us will smell and perceive it in a different way depending on genetic make-up, memory and a thousand other factors I am sure we have yet to discover.

To me, Clary Sage smells like cold tea. And for me, a cup of tea is the most comforting thing in the world (I am so very English, aren't

I?!) Is that why I perceive it that way I wonder? Clary Sage is cosy, warm and safe. To me, Clary Sage is a *cwtch.*

Do you know the word?

Locals say it a lot here in Ludlow, as does my sister working as a midwife in Wales. It is a Welsh word. (Ludlow is 10 minutes away from the England - Wales border.) Cwtch does not have a direct translation into English; its closest you and I might say is a hug or cuddle. But it means so much more than that. It means a safe place rested in someone's heart. It does have another meaning too, which is a closet or hiding place (perhaps under the stairs, for instance), and again it means "hidden somewhere safely and protected."

So yes, to me Clary Sage is a cwtch.

The moon connections are compassion, sympathy, empathy; our homeland, our mother land.

It is the rhythm of daily or family life as well as biological rhythms. It is connected to habits and instincts.

And whilst we won't say it is problems to do with the mother, it is very much about one's sense of belonging and where a person feels that they came from. So, it's a thread of blood lines and a sense of place. It makes me think of children who are searching for their biological parents or who have been ousted from their homes. These tortured souls desperate to leave Syria; that of their pain when the adrenaline drops and they find themselves on dry land dissected from all that they knew? (I only just realised the first thing that sprung to my mind was the homeland where Clary Sage originated. You tell me, that's not weird!) Where the connection is little more than a memory or even a whisper of a memory that might once have been, Clary Sage opens the door.

I think of how the moon's glow affects how I can see the garden at night, turning it sliver. Whilst I cannot see every part of the planting as I can in the sunlight, there is a soft outline that shows me where things start and end. Moon symbolism describes how our childhood experiences dictate the boundaries we have as adults. Are we soft and accepting like the moon's glow or are the walls we build hard and fortified with barbed wire?

Incidentally, these moon qualities seem to show themselves most of all when we are stressed. Those days when we want to stay at home and barricade the door. We find we want to sit quietly and simply be alone with ourselves (and actually, to *be* ourselves.). Then…the shadows are lifting just for a few hours and there is a moon glow through the clouds.

In "healthy" moon status, we see an easy flow of love between the person and their family, friends and humankind. They are rooted and have a good sense of their place in the world. But out of kilter we see psychosomatic illness and hypochondria. There are vast distortions of self image and tragically painful feelings of alienation from those around them.

Physically it's interesting to know that, in the context of Clary Sage, the moon governs the brain and the reproductive systems.

Mercury Medicine

Now interestingly as I said, Clary Sage has two ruling planets. It is also ruled by the planet of thought and communication; Mercury by its Roman name, Hermes by his Greek. Hermes was the son of Zeus and the brother of Apollo. He was a silver tongued devil, able to convince and persuade. He was extremely quick witted and a very clever merchant. He was however a liar and trickster. Even when he was the smallest infant he stole his brother, Apollo's, cattle. He ate some of them, sold the rest and then bare faced lied to Zeus when his father demanded "Where's the beef?"

It is worth recognising here, I think, that Zeus seems to have immediately known who the guilty party was likely to be. One does not earn that type of reputation overnight! Apollo leveraged his brother's misdemeanour for all it was worth. Hermes had created a beautiful lyre fashioned from a tortoise shell. Apollo forced Hermes to pay his debt to him and the lyre became Apollo's, giving him dominion over music (although Hermes is still considered the *father* of music). In return for the instrument, Apollo gave Hermes his caduceus, the magical staff wrapped in a serpent, the symbol of medicine and healing. As such Mercury is seen as the ruler of medicine. I like the fact that the term "Hermetic", which means "sealed" is now given to certain medical and laboratory procedures.

Mercury is attributed to being the father of mathematics, the alphabet, gymnastics, music and gambling.

You will often see mercury associated with commerce (and I suppose that has links with maths and gambling too!) but he is about quick dealing and fast paced economics. He makes me think of a really good sales person (and those of you who know me well will recognise that as the ultimate compliment, rather than an insult!) He says the right things, the correct things, he is persuasive and charismatic. And of course that is uber-sexy!

Often you can see him related to the court jester because he can say what he damn well pleases with a twinkle in his eye and a joke that will always be taken the right way. There might be a moment's stunned silence as everyone gasps at his audacity to have said something quite so outrageous and then people start to chuckle and contagiously gaffaw! (You might notice a familiar character here again, how was William Salmon described...?) Did you know that part of the court jester's role was to criticise the monarch, and they could get away with it because it was believed they "could not help it"? The jester was chosen for being a natural fool and as such, it was believed that his madness was divine. Either he was too stupid to know any better or he had a regal duty to tell the truth.

Think though of what Viola says about Feste the jester to Countess Olivia's household in Shakespeare's Twelfth Night

"This fellow is wise enough to play the fool;
And to do that well craves a kind of wit:
He must observe their mood on whom he jests,
The quality of persons, and the time,"

He's *wise* enough. *Not* stupid enough....

And she points out that he is very good at gauging people's moods. That thought has been bugging me for days, and you'll see why I think in a moment.

It's important too, to know that mercury is the messenger from the gods.

You might recall his winged helmet and sandals? These enabled him to travel unfettered, soaring up to the gods, down to commune with the mortals and then plummeting to the depths of the underworld taking messages from each. He is able to connect with all parts.

This reminds me of the theories of the eminent psychiatrist, Stanislav Grof. He hypothesised that consciousness seemed to come from the *universe* as opposed to being seated in the brain. So the

40

brain acts as a kind of *receiver* to ideas, rather than being the place where these ideas originate. It seems to me that mercury is like a kind of satellite dish gathering information from the gods and filtering it into the brain.

Grof distinguishes between two separate modes of consciousness. He calls these the *hylotropic* and the *holotropic*. The *hylotropic* mode pertains to how we experience "the normal, everyday experience of consensus reality" in other words...normality. By contrast the *holotropic* has to do with any state that aims at achieving wholeness and experiencing a totality of existence. This holotropic state would be best understood by we lay people as meditative, mystical, or psychedelic experiences, for example. (Much of his work was created by studying people on LSD) He terms these as "non-ordinary conscious states" and describes how contemporary psychiatry will often label these so called non-ordinary states as *psychotic.* With Grofs analogy of the brain being like a receiver, we then have to ask ourselves the very mercurial question...but do they indeed come from inside of the *brain* or from somewhere else entirely?

Grof uses the analogy that we can take wires out of a television set and it will *distort* the picture, but whilst that doesn't prove that the picture comes from outside, it does not prove that the picture originates from *inside* the set either. Similarly, he says, a scientist can alter consciousness by putting electrodes onto someone's head, but again, this does not prove that consciousness arose from inside brain. He felt these "experiences" **only disrupted the reception of a message that was coming through** and that could have come from anywhere. I suppose today's far greater leanings toward meditation might support this. That one learns to let go of fixed ideas and just let the thoughts pass through like "Clouds on an internal sky." Physically, we should note that mercury rules the eyes, the mucous membranes and the lungs. That is very Clary Sage-y too, isn't it?

Mercury and the Moon together...

Mercury and the moon have a lot in common. They are both very fast moving planets (although technically the moon is a satellite of the Earth, rather than a planet, of course) Where, metaphysically the moon represents our emotions, mercury represents our thoughts. I was interested to discover that Mercury does not have an atmosphere. If you were to stand on its surface you could see forever and ever, unlike the clouded perception you have from Earth. This is very much the essence of mercury too...this clear unclouded thinking.

The footsteps left by Neil Armstrong and Buzz Aldrin (I suppose I had better add "allegedly left" to keep the cynics happy!) will last in the moon's surface for thousands of years to come. But Mercury suffers no erosion at all, so if they had stood *there*, those footsteps would *never* fade, they would remain for all of eternity. Any event that mercury witnesses will be recorded for all of time. It will always be remembered. This is an important thing to recognise in mercury medicine...we are thinking about long term memory and the impact it has on the psyche. Mercurial plants are always our best friends here.

Now, normally I would not wander so far into the metaphysical realm but I found this fascinating. So then I wanted to know what it would represent when we experienced the moon/mercury archetype. How do the two planets affect each other? What's interesting is it fluctuates and changes. Mercury is a wonderful friend to the moon. Where the moon is about self image for example, mercury keeps the perception clear. We like how we look. We are happy that we are capable people who have value and deserve to be loved. However this relationship also has a negative aspect because the moon is not a good friend in return.

Where mercury rules friendships, the moon thinks she has outgrown them and often smashes them to pieces for no good reason. Mercury rules conversation but the moon does not listen to anyone else's point of view. All she is interested in is validating her own and if she perceives that she is not supported then she will cut the person off completely. There are arguments because she feels no-one is on her side. She feels isolated and alienated. There is no telling her to be reasonable either. She will jump to conclusions and irrationally seek everywhere for colluding evidence. If she thinks that her man may be cheating for instance, she'll be checking his phone, following him, if he doesn't answer his phone "He's with her", if he is late from work "He's with *her*". Our lady's thinking is entirely clouded by these beliefs that she must conclude is correct. Potentially she recognises that she is being a tiny bit mad too, but she simply cannot stop herself from doing it.

This really reminds me of something. It is as familiar to me as night and day. Do you feel a vague recognition too...?

Hold that thought.

We are leaving the ancient Greeks and Romans now, and heading to 21st century laboratories and hermetically sealed canisters containing....

Oestrogen

To recap...around about 5% of the chemical make up of Clary Sage is a component called sclareol which is said to have the same chemical structure as oestrogen. (Just in case you haven't noticed the very strange notion that the plant Hormium seems to affect hormones...) Aromatic experts then, propose that it mimics the effects of oestrogen in our body. If that were true, and so far I cannot find a clinical trial that definitively says it is...but if it were, what would that mean?

Well, we know it would help menstruation and menopause, and there are clinical trials that show that to be true. Loads of evidence....

But the world just became a clearer place to me...because scientists have recently begun to understand oestrogen on a far more intimate basis and the future, people, well frankly it is looking very hormonal indeed.

Oestrogen and its effects on reproduction

I'm going to start with reproductive science and work outwards from there because I think that's where most of us possess the most hormonal knowledge. I suspect all of us will recognise that oestrogen rises and falls during their menstrual cycle and also through our female lives. Incidentally, men also have oestrogen, which is synthesized from testosterone, but during a woman's fertile life, her levels are significantly higher than a man's.

So...this is a bird's eye view down onto oestrogenic fluctuations throughout our lives.

Oestrogen influences the changes we see in puberty, pregnancy, birth and menopause and also is involved in premenstrual bodily activities. It is produced in the ovaries and is regulated by the pituitary gland. In our fertile lives, it causes ova to mature and then thickens the lining of the womb. In pregnancy the levels go up and then fall rapidly after birth. It is thought that this fall in hormones may be the cause of postnatal depression. As the ovaries diminish during the perimenopause the production of oestrogen falls. As the ovaries cease during menopause, oestrogen production ceases.

To put this into context, let's just quickly remind ourselves of the other hormones involved in the process.

These are:

Gonadotrophin Releasing Hormone (GnRH)

This is manufactured in the hippothalamus. It is secreted to trigger FSH

Luteinising Hormone (LH)

Again this is secreted by the pituitary, and it ripens the follicles ready to be released at ovulation.

Follicle Stimulating Hormone FSH

Releases a matured egg in what you and I recognise as ovulation

Progesterone

Progesterone is also produced in the ovaries and in the placenta too. When an egg is released from the ovaries, it travels down the fallopian tubes but its follicle is left behind. We call this empty shell the corpus luteal. This then disintegrates and begins to secrete progesterone too. For optimum fertility levels the body requires a corpus luteal phase of around 10 days, any shorter and the lining of the womb does not have enough strength to maintain a pregnancy.

Again progesterone levels fall rapidly after pregnancy, potentially causing postal depression.

This cycle continues throughout our lives until the ovarian pool is exhausted and menopause begins.

But the cessation of the period might not be entirely in line with the last few eggs, which can explain why some late life pregnancies can catch women unawares.

Those final few months of perimenopause are critical to understanding the symptoms connected with it. Here symptoms happen, not because of depleted oestrogen (usually!) but instead there is an oestrogen dominant environment. The ovaries are secreting oestrogen but not every cycle will release and egg and so therefore there is a deficit in the corpus luteal to make progesterone. Ergo there is more oestrogen than progesterone.

Then as menopause happens, oestrogen disappears....

So periods are over (Thank, heavens above!)

But what else?

So far we know of about 400 different functions that oestrogen is involved in, throughout the body. (I'm glad I don't have to resit my Anatomy and Physiology papers now!) So when these oestrogen levels fall, it impacts the body in more ways than you can possibly imagine. I suspect that we are all going to be petrified by these new findings and so every now and then I am going to whisper some reassurance into your ear as you read...

Clary Sage....

Hopefully that will prevent too many tears on your book, but I can't guarantee it, girls.

Other functions of Oestrogen

Here is a list of what oestrogen does, above and beyond its well known effects on the reproductive life.

• Increases and piques sexual interest

• Enhances energy

• Increases the rate of metabolism

• Improves our sensitivity to insulin

In the tissues it:

- Maintains bone density
- Protects us against muscle damage
- Regulates our body temperature
- Maintains muscular tissue
- Reduces the risk we have of developing cataracts as well as preventing macular degeneration
- Maintains the amount of collagen in the skin, maintains elasticity and reduces wrinkling
- The thickness and softness of the skin is determined by oestrogen as is the amount of water contained within
- It also guards against tooth loss

Effects on the heart

- Oestrogen protects our hearts against strokes and heart disease.

- Maintains elasticity in the walls of the arteries and also dilates smaller arteries. It keeps arteries open by acting as a natural calcium channel blocker.

- It binds to receptors in the endothelium and oestrogen stimulates the release of nitric oxide that then causes vasodilation.

- It reduces levels of homocysteine, the amino acid that thickens the blood and causes clotting.

- It prevents blood platelets from becoming too sticky.

- It improves blood flow throughout the body and in particular the vessels of the heart. This of course also reduces blood pressure.

- Reduces the amount of plaque accumulating on the arteries

- It acts upon cholesterol

- Reduces harmful LDL cholesterol and stops it from oxidising, as well as increasing the healthy cholesterol (HDL) by as much as 10-15%

- Overall the presence of oestrogen decreases a person's risk of heart disease by a massive 40% to 50%.

Belly Fat

When I was in Beijing I listened to a brilliant talk by Dr Marilyn Glenville about fat around the middle and how it leads to illnesses such as diabetes (which I knew) as well as many other illnesses such as Alzheimer's Disease (which I didn't). Apparently there is a school of thought that says Alzheimer's should be renamed Diabetes Type III because the actions on the brain are exactly the same as happens to the pancreas.

Later we'll look at Poly Cystic Ovarian Syndrome in more detail but here I just want to draw your attention to the fact that about 40% of women with PCOS are overweight.

The terrifying thing is that the fat in their bellies actually starts acting like an organ on its own…and starts making even more oestrogen. Although we don't know why that is, it is interesting to learn that *men* with low levels of oestrogen develop larger bellies and again then we start to see the related health concerns.

What happens to the waistline after menopause gals? It certainly isn't so easy to keep neat and trim, is it ladies? And the reason for this is the dwindling levels of oestrogen.

That would be impressive enough, wouldn't it? But research at the turn of the century uncovered two most extraordinary pieces of information about oestrogen.

Firstly, that is neuroprotective.

And the second...? Well... I save that for the next chapter if that's ok with you.

Neurological

It is recognised that certain mental disorders are more prevalent in men than women, such as schizophrenia and autism for example, and that anxiety, depression and PTSD are more prevalent in women and until recently it seemed impossible to determine why that might be.

Schizophrenia for instance has an onset stage of four years earlier in men than women, but there seems to be a second surge in women between the ages of 45-54. If women do develop schizophrenia it is relatively mild, unless menopause has taken place and then symptoms can be profoundly severe.

Alzheimer's is a severe form of dementia that is between 33-66% more likely to happen to women. The fact that we have the generation of baby boomers in old people's homes and also the increased life span on the society as a whole still does not seem enough to explain why this illness would affect so many more women than men.

Possibly the 21st Century's biggest gift to medicine is its investigations into the cognitive functions for oestrogen. (How strange that it should come at at time when the planet is becoming more in tune with its feminine side.)

We now know that oestrogen influences brain function through receptors on neurons in multiple areas of the brain as well as throughout the body. There are in fact two different types of receptor and four types of oestrogen, but the sakes of simplicity for this book, we will simply address them as one, as oestrogen as a whole.

Scientists have discovered that it protects, against oxidative stress, ischemic injury (adverse events of the blood supply to the heart), hypoglycemic injury (adverse events in the body's blood sugar mechanisms) and also the amyloid protein which is suspected to be at the root of the progression of Alzheimer's Disease.

It stimulates production of the nerve growth factors which means that not only does it protect the nerves but it also helps to replace any damaged ones too.

Remember what a synapse is from your Nervous System lessons? It is the electrical message that crosses between nerves. Well, at a synapse oestrogen actually increases how concentrated the amounts of serotonin, norepinephrine (or you might know that as noradrenaline) and dopamine are. It affects their release, their uptake and also their activation.

Most importantly oestrogen increases the number of receptors for these neurotransmitters to activate. Just take a moment to think about that for a second. If oestrogen drops them there are less places for happiness ligands to grab onto, what is going to happen?

Low mood right?

So think of the oestrogen drop we experience as our period approaches, the post natal blues and the depression we associate with menopause....

Now this is where it gets interesting / terrifying depending on your viewpoint.

We know that oestrogen affects blood flow, not just from the obvious monthly clue, but also from our notes about how it affects the heart. Now, when the body requires more strength (for fight and flight, for instance, in stress) it moves blood flow away from unnecessary systems. (Think of how your shiver when you are scared. One of the reasons is because the blood has been drained from the skin to feed more important systems in the fight). But the brain cannot do this. It needs all the blood it can get and in fact 2/3rds of the brain is made up of blood vessels. Actually, as yet we do not know how blood perfusion in the brain is affected but common thought is it is safe to suggest it mimics the actions on the heart, which have been extensively studied. (To repeat: the oestrogen receptors in the endothelium then stimulate the release of nitric oxide which causes vasodilation)

Now...

A recent trial examined the vasodilatory effects of oestrogen on the brain using an ultrasound. They discovered that post menopausal women had less cerebral flow than those who were premenopausal. Indeed, when they supplemented them with oestrogen replacement therapy (ERT Yeah, yeah, I l know oestrogen doesn't start with E! Score one nil for the US spelling police!) the cerebral flow improved. By two months into the treatment it was significantly improved and it continued to improve throughout the 52 weeks of the rest of the trial.

But now here it gets very unsettling indeed, and I'd ask you to remember this research is so young it can hardly crawl yet, let alone walk, but...

Oestrogen's affect on the bodymind
Oestrogen receptors are found throughout the bodymind, in the places we might suspect, like the womb etc, but they are also found in the brain, most especially in the limbic system. They are found in several places including the amygdala and the hippothalamus.

Now just for fun, see if you can remember the functions of the hippothalamus.....

The two I was hoping you might remember are *storage of memories* and also *regulation of temperature,* but you could also have had regulating thirst, hunger, sleep, mood or sex drive or if you were a proper A & P swot you might have gone the whole hog and said maintains homeostasis, which would have taken you to the top of the class.

But for this particular horror story we need to remember two things....that the storage of memories and temp are involved and unlike other systems in the body which have evolved to be able to borrow from other areas in times of crisis, remember that the brain needs all of its blood flow. I'm going to apologise before I move on because I know a great number of us are going to become upset and scared by the next section.

Hot Flushes

85% of perimenopausal women experience hot flushes (I think gals call them hot flashes) and it is now thought these originate from the brain and that they are directly related to hypoestrogenism (low oestrogen).

It now seems that hot flushes might not simply be symptoms of the menopause, but there is gathering evidence that they may actually *cause* the cerebral deterioration into Alzheimer's. Tests show that there is reduced blood flow to the brain during a hot flush and the greatest change of flow was seen in the hippothalamus. These patterns of regional flow are very similar to how Alzheimer's presents. Again when the ladies were supplemented with ERT the hot flushes improved. Reproductive researchers now assert that hot flushes eventually lead to degenerative damage to the brain and in fact these vasoconstrictive moments resemble how plaque forms on the heart and arteries. The hippothalamus is so damaged that neurons can no longer repair it and so we see this devastating memory loss. (Just as an aside this really made me think back to the rose book and how rose oil can assist the plasticity –repair- of cells in the hippothalamus in early onset dementia so maybe not all is lost…)

Clary Sage…

Now, men's cognition tends to deteriorate a good decade later than women's and this is due to what's known as aromatization of oestrogen (and strangely that has nothing at all to do with fragrance!) This is the way enzymes change testosterone into oestrogen. By their sixties, men have almost three times as much oestrogen than women of the same age because *their* levels don't decline and researchers feel this probably the reason for the far higher incidence rate of Alzheimer's in women than men. It's all terribly sad, isn't it? And more than a little frightening.

As you would imagine, studies into oestrogen and cognitive processing are now widespread however it can be very hard to draw exact conclusions from them because the drop out rates of the trials can be skewed by the fact that those people themselves may have poor cognitive processing but...it seems very likely that the link between estrogen and cognition is particularly between verbal memory (which is our recollection of words) and verbal reasoning (which in the simplest terms is our ability to think constructively).

I drew a completely unsubstantiated parallel, in my head, with the molecule Tribolone. This is a synthetic molecule given by oral administration to menopausal women suffering from related symptoms. It is converted into three different metabolites, each of which had oestrogenic effects. The 2006 paper states:

Tibolone seems to be effective on estrogen-withdrawal symptoms such as hot flushes, sweating, insomnia, headache, and vaginal dryness, with results generally comparable to the effects exerted by estrogen-based treatments, and the additional property of a progestogenic activity on the endometrium. As well as relieving vasomotor symptoms, tibolone has positive effects on sexual well-being and mood, and improves dyspareunia and libido. These effects may depend on both estrogenic and androgenic actions exerted at the genital level and in the central nervous system, and on a reduction of sex-hormone-binding globulin and an increase of free testosterone, without affecting Δ-5 androgens levels."

So we have to ask ourselves...without clinical evidence that sclareol is acting on oestrogenic receptors, can we believe that Clary Sage could do the same? I have found nothing to convince me that they would not. And I don't think it hurts to emulate the likes of Dioscorides and Culpepper, to observe and follow the clues. For me the clues say, it probably does.

Chemical effects of Oestrogen

Earlier I stated there were over 400 effects but have listed very few so far so now let's have a look at what they think oestrogen does to the neurochemistry of the body

It increases the levels of norepinephrine in the body

If you don't remember- norepinephrine (or noradrenaline) is the stress hormone that shuts down all the other processes in the body to ensure you have enough resources to fight or flight. Then, it quickens the breathing, ups the heart rate, redirects the blood sugar and then super charges the brain with oxygen. It can do this because digestion and growth systems have "donated" their power at its request.

Without oestrogen to keep norepinephrine topped up not only do we struggle to cope with stress, but our emotional and physical energy reserves begin to suffer too. (Incidentally it is thought this might be why women can multitask and deal with stressful situations better than men can – the high oestrogen helps them to coast.)

Decreases dopamine release;

Now, dopamine is known to be in control of our learning and reward systems in the body, and much was made of this discovery in the media, because it impacts on stress but also addiction too. But recently it has been discovered that dopamine is more concerned with the *expectation* of a reward.

For example, Wolfram Schulz originally pioneered the first experiment that gave us real insights into what dopamine did in the 1990's. He monitored neurons from brain cells when a dog was given a taste of juice after a light had come on. He switched on the bulb, delivered the juice and then the dopamine cells would fire. This is where the reward theory came from. But then over time, dogs being the intelligent creatures they are, when the light came on the beast went for the juice, gulped it down and enjoyed it...but the dopamine stopped firing.

Around about the same time, another set of psychological experiments were happening involving computer systems. They wanted to investigate trial and error and they surmised that learning takes place when events are unexpected. Their software could do many different things include playing a game of backgammon! Their algorithm relied on what is called "prediction error" in other words the difference between what you expect and then what you actually get.

These two studies and many more, still undergoing, are altering our perception of precisely what dopamine does. It closely monitors what reactions we expect when we predict things (based on our own human experience and history) and then releases its neurotransmitters based on that.

Oestrogen is involved in producing neurotrophic factors.
 These are a group of proteins which are involved in maintaining cell health, helping them to grow and replacing damaged ones. We can call them Brain Fertiliser, really! It is recognised that these have a direct bearing on depression.

It increases both brain and blood stream levels of endorphins
So low levels would mean you have a poorer resistance to pain. They are, of course, at their highest when you go into labour.

Oestrogen is involved in the production of allopregnanolone and also to has an indirect effect on DHEA

These "neurosteroid" relationships are desirable because they both are very good at reducing anxiety levels.

It has many effects on serotonin, including an effect on tryptophan levels in the blood which is the amino acid that synthesizes into serotonin. To cut a very long endocrine story short when the levels of oestrogen drop we become anxious, afraid and depressed and if we did have a natural oestrogen, we could up the levels of our mood moderator, serotonin.

It may possibly have a relationship with melatonin

The connection with the sleep-regulating hormone is still unverified because every animal has a slightly different structure here so experiments are not easy to do . It is however believed to have a very strong relationship.

What we do know, of course, is that Clary Sage will definitely help you to sleep, it will reduce anxiety and it will also alleviate symptoms of depression.

Other functions of oestrogen that might be relevant here are:

It enhances production of nerve-growth factor

It improves mood and increases concentration

• It improves uptake of magnesium, our natural tranquilizer

• Helps maintain memory

• Increases reasoning and new ideas

• Improves fine motor skills (next time you are premenstrual watch how many more things you drop and trip over)

• And of course, it improves sleep

Oestrogen and Fear

So if that wasn't hard enough for you to read, I'm going to take us even further into hell.

After several millennia of women bleeding and everyone marveling at her becoming like the devil incarnate incredibly finally, there are some insights about why this might be.

Welcome to what might be the most powerful of the molecules of emotion.

It is now believed that oestrogen helps us to deal with fear and more specifically a psychological concept called Fear Extinction, which I'll explain in a moment.

Let's close our eyes and try it on for size.

Might we become the Goddess of Destruction because we are more afraid and anxious as the oestrogen drops...? I have always felt that the arguments I have when I am premenstrual are the same annoyances I have the rest of the month, I just feel them more acutely.

It feels right to me.

Does it to you?

Let's explore it a bit more.

We have already said that women are more likely to suffer from illnesses such as anxiety, depression and Post Traumatic Stress Disorder than men. Indeed there is usually an element of anxiety involved in depression and vice versa, and of course PTSD is usually some kind of combination of all three.

So scientists wondered at that. Why would women suffer PTSD more often than men, have more acute symptoms and suffer it for longer? It is suspected that their traumatic events may have co-incided with the hormonal fluctuations in their cycle. So...if a bomb went off for our Afghanistan veteran (give the heroine of our Sweet Basil book a wave, this is a hard moment for her) and she had already ovulated then she might not have adequate oestrogenic resources to deal with the fear that she would have done at the beginning of the month and because of the hormonal levels she is not able to extinguish the fear.

Fear Extinction

Fear Extinction is defined as a decline in conditioned fear responses. Do we remember Pavlov's dogs? Pavlov conditioned the dogs to salivate when he rang a bell, because they would get food. Then after a while he took away the food, but for a while their canine conditioned minds thought dog treats were imminent and so they continued to drool at the thought of it. After a period of time though, they sussed the ruse and the conditioning was extinguished. No more slobber. This paradigm shows us how we learn behavior and more importantly how our brain remembers and processes it.

After many thousands of hours of lab time across the planet it has been mapped that the fear conditioning happens across the hippocampus, the amygdala and the ventromedial pre frontal cortex. Then in 2012 a paper was published that will change the entire face of mental health. Lebron-Miland and Miland's paper *"Sex differences, gonadal hormones and the fear extinction network: implications for anxiety disorders"* proposed that oestrogen was fundamental to the fear extinction network. In other words that memories would fade, or new ones could be more easily overlaid if there was oestrogen present. Post doctoral research by The Ebony Institute born this out, that the higher the level of oestrogen was in a woman's blood, the less likely she was to startle. In fact in both rat and human studies, researchers have been able to conclude that the response to a neutral trigger will be less fearful when oestrogen levels are high.

Most interestingly in a study of women who had suffered a sexual attack, those women who had taken the morning after pill suffered far lesser effects of PTSD than those who had not (although the brand with the most success was an oestrogen/progesterone combi pill).

I can't help but think it is such a cruel twist of fate that meant their menstrual cycle was in a place to dictate that she could not erase the memory and fear of her crisis. Now it means that she cannot relearn and imagine that that fear does not live outside of the door. Too little oestrogen means too little dopamine to train her brain to expect a difference.

Clary Sage...

To cut an extremely long story short, it has been found that supplementing men with ERT can also help Obsessive Compulsive Disorder. (How about that for moon medicine that rules habits and instincts!) The ramifications for this new understanding of fear seem to be endless for researchers trying to find better ways to treat psychosis and schizophrenia.

So...I tried not to be too long winded but I think I failed, but Clary Sage was an important medicine that has helped in childbirth, anxiety, sleep disorders and menopause and where we weren't really sure why...we are not only getting an understanding of how the plant world has possibly far out-evolved us, but also some vitally important ways to use aromatherapy that potentially will outstrip the orthodox medical profession.

There's only one problem...

There's no evidence that Clary Sage *does* mimic oestrogen.

Oh that old chestnut! We've been alright so far haven't we!

Omega 3

I can't write a book about Clary Sage without mentioning *Clary Sage Seed Oil* which is a different product from our distilled essential oil but still clearly comes from our gorgeous plant.

In aromatherapy we use an oil which is distilled from the flowering tops and the leaves. There is, however, a fabulous supplement on the market of Clary Sage *seed* oil. (Remember both Culpepper and Dioscorides both had great things to say about the seeds but we cannot leverage these with the e/o.)

To make it even more confusing it is called Essential Oil too, but here we are referring to essential fatty acids, rather than our distilled bottle of gorgeousness.

This is an Omega 3 supplement. In fact it is the strongest and most stable supplement of its kind on the market. I am indebted to Robert Tisserand for unknotting my thinking because I was trying to work out evidence that Omega 3 would not be in the e/o. He gently and patiently reminded me that Omega 3 only exists in cold pressed oils and so could only be in the seed oil. (Thank you Robert, my poor brain was beginning to hurt!)

I talk about Omega 3 extensively in my Bronchitis book and the benefits of using it after trauma, because it balances out the effects of omega 6 which is pro-inflammatory. The interesting thing about omega 3 though, is our bodies do not manufacture it naturally. It has to come from food. Where previously it had been thought that fish oils and flax seed were the best sources of this, it seems that Clary Sage seed oil may be a big contender for that place. I am a bit disappointed to find you can only buy it in capsules though, because how great would that have been to use as a carrier oil?!

The research in this area is very new and it is being very aggressively pushed by an Israeli doctor, Dr. Adiel Tel-Oren MD. He speaks a great deal about the benefits on Youtube and he is mesmerizing to watch. He is erudite and well informed. The funny thing is that the internet is full of people questioning *his* background. A page on the Jerusalem post warns:

The Health Ministry issued a warning yesterday about a man named Adiel Tel-Oren who presents himself as a physician but is an imposter. He is "unlicensed to practice medicine in Israel. He treats patients in his clinic while using preparations that are liable to endanger health and are not approved for use," the ministry said on Thursday.

Looks like mercurial medicine has captured another William Salmon to its bidding, doesn't it?!

In balance, the Post then reports:

Dr. Tel Oren's office said in response: "Dr. Adiel Tel Oren never presented himself as a doctor in Israel, despite his education and qualifications in medicine, and he certainly was not an imposter physician. Dr. Tel Oren does not give medical treatments that require a medical license from the Health Ministry, but rather alternative holistic skin treatments. Hundreds of patients who gave up on conventional medicine can testify to the success of his treatments, which alleviated their conditions."

300 years after William Salmon, conventional medicine is still proclaiming quack doctors and Mountebacks and clary Sage is still drawing these people to her service

What a very strange world healing is.

Anyway, let's have a look at what the "real" doctors have to say about their findings into Clary Sage

Clinical Evidence into Clary Sage

Anxiolytic

An extremely interesting trial was published by Ariel University in Israel about the insights they had gained into how Clary Sage exerted an anxiolytic effect. Just as a recap the word that would make me fail any spelling bee, *anxiolytic* means reducing anxiety. They found that it contained twice as much omega 3 any other species of sage (so although they say Clary Sage, we have to assume they are using the *seed* oil here) and that these affected a series of pathways called *eicosanoid synthesis pathways.*

These are one of the most complex systems in the body and they are concerned with bringing the body back into homeostasis.

They kick into action during:

- During growth
- After physical activity and exertion
- When there is inflammation in the body
- When our body uses immunity
- If we consume some kind of toxic compound or pathogen

So we can say these pathways are serious warriors on our behalf. They are the defenders.

Now this pathway requires omega 3 and omega 6 to function effectively. The omegas synthesize into eicosanoids which then act as the signalling molecules which you and I recognize as hormones. There are several types of eicosanoids including *prostaglandins, thromboxanes, leukotrienes, lipoxins* and *eoxins.*

So what does each do?

Prostaglandins

- They control inflammation
- Blood flow
- Formation of clots
- Uterine contractions in labour

(C'mon, tell me you are not excited to see the last one…it's the omega 3 on the eicosanoids ladies!)

Thomboxanes

As you might guess, named for its role in clot formation (think thrombosis) and it is an enzyme in blood platelets.

Leukotrienes, lipoxins and eoxins:

Are all pro-inflammation markers and have also been found in immunity cells.

Because they rely on Omega 3, then Clary Sage is like double dosing and so ramps up the action.

Now, this trial made me think of a recent trip to take a friend to show her where to buy some CS. The lady behind the counter said "Clary Sage always makes me think of the pregnant ladies who come in to buy it..."

Yep, we'd all agree that we want wee babba out as fast as we can so I think we would all go to maternity equipped but...

Listen to this.

The trial tells of pregnant ratties who were given an oil based supplement to their feed. The massive munchers either had Clary Sage oil or sunflower oil as the placebo.

Guess what?

The baby ratties all showed less dominant behavior and less anxiety like traits right up to the end of the trial at 3 months of age....

The *babies* are calmer....

They were more submissive and their blood cortisol levels were lower.

The offspring don't just emerge more easily, they are scientifically proven to be more relaxed rodents!

Lovin' it!!!

Just in case you are a midwife or an expectant mum, you can find that trial here: http://www.aromaticscience.com/chronic-food-administration-of-salvia-sclarea-oil-reduces-animals-anxious-and-dominant-behavior/

If you are dealing with having babies, then I suggest you read this fab article on a study of women in labour at Oxford Brookes University, which cites CS in their tool kit. Here they describe how Clary Sage makes labour shorter and less painful.

http://www.independent.co.uk/life-style/health-and-families/health-news/epidural-all-i-need-is-rose-oil-737976.html

Dopamine

Now, this time our rats were asked to swim. Erm, ok, it was an FST, so they were Forced to swim. And I would like to tell you that had sniffed CS, but no, they had it injected interperitoneally...apart from that it is all good!

Anyway they were treated with a different essential oil in turn, Roman Camomile, Rosemary, Clary Sage and Lavender. By far the most effective anti-stressor for the rats was Clary Sage (at 5%). Here using various agonists and antagonists they were then able to tell us that the reason is because Clary Sage also acts on the dopaminergic pathways. Again, they suggested that this is more evidence for investigating Clary Sage further as a treatment for depression.

Cortisol and Serotonin

A beautiful clinical trial was conducted at Sookmyung Women's University in Seoul to look at how Clary Sage would affect cortisol and serotonin levels. Clearly this is fundamentally important data to use because it gives us tangible evidence of how the body is able to fight stress (through the cortisol) and also maintain mood (though 5-HT serotonin)

Here, 22 menopausal women were chosen in their 50's although it gives no real explanation as to why this group were chosen. They were divided into two groups as having normal and depressive states and they were monitored and gauged using two Depression Inventory Scales. (These are the Korean versions of the Beck Inventory Scales do KBDI 1 & 2.)

In both groups the cortisol levels were reduced significantly (by 31% according to the KBDI 2 and 16% scoring by the KBDI 1 and also Thyroid Stimulating Hormone was decreased too, although not by a huge amount. The exciting part was how much it elevated the mood.

In the "normal" group

Gauging by the KBDI- 1, an increase of 5-HT of 341%

Gauging by the KBDI- 2, an increase of 5-HT of 828%

In the depressed group

Gauging by the KBDI- 1, an increase of 5-HT of 484%

Gauging by the KBDI- 2, an increase of 5-HT of 257%

I am guessing then that the longer a depressed person uses clary sage, the more powerful the effects will become, because when they are poorly it makes them feel as much as 5 times better but when they are on top of things we are looking at as much a 9 times better still.

(No wonder those baby rats were chilled...life feels seriously *good* man!)

http://www.aromaticscience.com/changes-in-5-hydroxytryptamine-and-cortisol-plasma-levels-in-menopausal-women-after-inhalation-of-clary-sage-oil/

Dysmenorrhea:

There is a lovely trial by Dr Jane Buckle done on college students. Because it also includes lavender and rose it can tell us very little about the actions of Clary Sage, except that it reduced the severity of their menstrual cramps.

It is useful however to know that she uses 2 drops lavender, 1 drop Clary Sage and 1 drop rosa centifolia in 5cc (that's a teaspoon to the rest of us) of almond oil.

http://www.aromaticscience.com/effect-of-aromatherapy-on-symptoms-of-dysmenorrhea-in-college-students-a-randomized-placebo-controlled-clinical-trial/

In Hungkuang University, Taichung, Taiwan, they took these findings a little further, left out rose and substituted marjoram. So their recipe was 1 drop of marjoram, 1 drop Clary Sage, 2 drops lavender. They worked more like I do in that they blended theirs into a blank moisturizer. Now this trial is interesting because most trials only ask the participants to massage during menstruation. This trial asked them to rub the cream into the abdomen from the last day of their period up to the first day of the next one.

Again the results saw a big decrease in pain scores but also the participants said that the pain went much quicker. Where previously they had been in pain for 2.4 days, their pain had disappeared in 1.8. (Incidentally we know from the findings of the rose book that the effects are cumulative and so next cycle we would expect that the pain would be for a shorter period still…no pun intended!)

http://www.ncbi.nlm.nih.gov/pubmed/22435409

Incidentally, if you do need any more help with period pains there is a gorgeous paper here:

http://www.phytotherapyjournal.com/File_Folder/33-
36(phytotherapy).pdf It is not relevant enough to Clary Sage to
discuss here, but if this doesn't get students an A+ in their case
histories nothing will! It's full of diet, nutrition, all manner of
goodies.

Wound Healing

Very quickly in Feb 2014, the University of Lodz revealed that Clary
Sage had been effective in eradicating pathogens of *Staphylococcus
aureus, S. epidermidis* and *S. xylosus*, all of which are problematic
infections for wound healing. To me, I think it makes best sense to
squirt with a blast of clary sage hydrolat, but just cleaning a wound
with a drop of clary sage on a cold compress seems sensible too.

http://www.ncbi.nlm.nih.gov/pubmed/25821423

Anti fungal

More for me and my ever growing file of attacks against moulds
that can cause breathing problems than for any of you....!

Marin et al. 2008

Clary Sage showed fungicidal activity against

- Aspergillus,

- Penicillium

- Fusarium species

- Trichoderma viride

- Mucor mucedo

- Aspergillus viride,

- Candida albicans,

- Bifonazole

- Cladosporium cladosporioides

- Trichophyton menthagrophytes

- Cladosporium fulvum

- Alternaria alternata,

- Phomopsis helianthi,

- Phoma macdonaldii

Clearly, this is useful to know for any yeast infections, but most obviously Candida.

http://www.doiserbia.nb.rs/Article.aspx?ID=0354-46640802233D&AspxAutoDetectCookieSupport=1#.VkM1TrfhAgs

Cancer

The next trial is fascinating because although it talks about tumours, it relates to that as a secondary action. Here, sadly our rats have been given tumours and then are injected with sclareol to see how it affects it. The clary sage reduces Interleukin 4 which is an inflammatory marker that shows itself when immunity drops. Here the paper explains that the tumour decreased in size but also the immune system was improved and so the paper concludes there is evidence to support further investigations into the idea of using it as a way to boost immunity in people undergoing cancer treatment.

Again, because the letters still find their way to my inbox about cancer treatment, I will stress...

So far neither orthodox medicine nor alternative medicine has yet found a treatment for cancer. But since we know that serotonin affects the chemotaxis of Tumour Necrosis Factor, diffusing essential oils may help to boost levels and improve their immunity and prospects in their fight against the disease. Lifting the spirits never hurt anyone.

http://www.aromaticscience.com/sclareol-reduces-cd4-cd25-foxp3-treg-cells-in-a-breast-cancer-model-in-vivo-2/

Breast cancer:

I suppose this small passage is the crux of the book really, isn't it? Not from the point of view of finding an essential oil that cures cancer because as you know so far no such cure has been found...only certain oils that will kills cells in a petri dish which sadly is a long way from being the same thing.

But, given that scientists believe that oestrogens can cause breast cancer from things like plastic containers...do we really want to be putting an essential oil onto our body with these components?

As ever the best person to consult about safety is Robert Tisserand and he answers that question in his blog post "is Clary Sage estrogenic"

"Sclareol does have an interesting anticancer activity, including in vitro *action against human breast cancer MCF-7 cells (Dimas et al 2006). An isomer, 13-epi-sclareol, which is also present in clary sage oil, inhibits the growth of breast and uterine cancers in* vitro, *and was slightly more potent than Tamoxifen, but was not toxic to normal cells (Sashidhara et al 2007). This suggests the possibility that sclareol might actually inhibit estrogen, and might after all have some capacity to interact with estrogen receptor sites.* **What we do know is that sclareol will not give you breast cancer."**

If you don't already follow RT's work, I would suggest that anyone with even the slightest interest in essential oils should do so and you can find his blog here. Sign up today: http://roberttisserand.com/2010/04/is-clary-sage-oil-estrogenic/

Despite the evidence he cites though, every bit of information I have found says that it must work with oestrogen. I would be very surprised if ultimately we find that it only *inhibits* rather than balances or promotes oestrogen.

Endothelial dysfunction

I wanted to end on this note because as regular readers of my work will know, I am fascinated by the molecule of Nitric Oxide (NO). It is though it has a close alignment with aggression and with pleasure. When we are pleasured (whether emotionally or physically) cells become flooded with NO. When there is too little NO then we become aggressive (very over simplistic but you catch my drift).

Incidentally remember from the list of actions earlier, we also know that *oestrogen* also encourages the flow of NO and when its levels drop then the heart has more difficulties, as do the lungs and actually the penis too...because it becomes harder to obtain and erection (no pun intended!)

Because I am that lazy to quote from my own Bronchitis book:

[Nitric oxide] is found in the tissues of every cell and so there is nowhere in our system that is more than one micron away from a supply of it. Its state as a gas means it can move through the body at a startling speed, far faster than many other neurotransmitters.

Its job, very simplistically speaking, is to smooth tissues. It plays a massive part in the cardiovascular and nervous systems. It is now also understood to play a fundamental part in immunity. It is found in the endothelial tissues (the lining) of each cell and it signals vascular smooth cells to relax so vasodilation can take place. Veins and arteries are filled with this relaxant gas and as Nitric Oxide (NO) is activated, it triggers blood vessels to open, allowing parts of the body to be better supplied with circulation.

Let's end with the Korean researcher's words from 2014:

Clary sage treatment of rats subjected to immobilization stress contributed to their recovery from endothelial dysfunction by increasing NO production and eNOS level as well as by decreasing oxidative stress. Appropriate concentration of clary sage may result in recovery from endothelial dysfunction. These findings indicate that clary sage oil may be effective in the prevention and treatment of stress-induced cardiovascular diseases.

http://www.ncbi.nlm.nih.gov/pubmed/25311097

Vibrational Medicine of Clary Sage

Looking though ancient healing books there is a resounding theme… dreams.

Use it for bad dreams, recurring dreams and also for encouraging insightful dreams.

It brings old, forgotten dreams back to the fore and as such we can find it motivating.

It helps one let go of worry.

We'll take that a step further and say it is calming to paranoia and hysteria.

It is euphoric and in the right circumstance, aphrodisiac.

Thinking of her plant signature with pink/ purple and violet flowers we can see she would vibrate on the chakras of the same colours. Certainly we would expect to see the brow chakra and indeed ancient usage does put Clary Sage as one of the most useful oils to meditate with for insights. (Very mercurial indeed!) This will also apply for dreams naturally. It should go without saying that the brow/pineal chakra is fundamentally connected with the brain and also the production of melatonin….

And the carousel comes round to the same spot again!

The pink resonates with the heart chakra, again quintessentially linked with emotions but also the respiratory system and Clary Sage is fantastic for breathing problems as well as the chest and breasts.

I'd be tempted to use it as root and sacral chakra medicine too, if there were issues about childhood history and "where have I come from?" as well as trauma from sexual assault.

Clary Sage Essential Oil

Fragrance

Cold tea!

I find that different sources can smell very different, where sometimes you might get a very spicy note, others might smell very herbaceous.

Note

Middle or heart note

Blends With

Citrus, woody and earthy tones.

Extraction

Steam distillation from flowering tops and leaves

Clary Sage in Aromatherapy

Actions are:

- Anticonvulsive
- Antidepressant
- Antiphlogistic – Reduces inflammation
- Antiseptic
- Antispasmodic
- Anti tussive

- Aphrodisiac – stops coughing

- Astringent

- Bactericidal

- Carminative

- Cicatrisant – helps form scar tissue

- Deodorant

- Digestive

- Emmenagogue – Brings on menstruation

- Hypotensive

- Nervine

- Sedative

- Stomachic

- Tonic

- Uterine

Use for:

- Amenorrhea – Absence of periods

- Dysmenorrhea – Painful periods

- Leucorrhoea   - White vaginal discharge

- Labour pains

- High blood pressure

- Muscular aches and pains

- Restless legs

- Asthma

- Throat infections
- Bronchitis
- Coughs inc. whooping cough
- Colic
- Dyspepsia
- Cramps
- Flatulence
- Acne
- Dandruff
- Boils and ulcers
- Oily skin
- Greasy hair
- Wrinkles
- Depression
- Frigidity
- Impotence
- Migraine
- Nervous tension
- Stress related disorders.

Excellent fragrance fixative in soaps and perfumery. The fragrance industry are also researching the possibility of synthesizing sclareol as a way of making a natural replacement to amber and ambergris fragrance notes.

Clary Sage in Practical Aromatherapy

There are two famous speeches from the Shakespeare's Hamlet. The first is in the graveyard when the Prince of Denmark lifts the exhumed skull and mock "Alas, poor Yorrick. I knew him, Horatio" of the court jester he remembered from his childhood. And then we have:

"To be, or not to be. That is the question".

To be, or not to be using Clary Sage....because there is contradiction everything we read. Here are some thoughts then.

Poly Cystic Ovarian Syndrome

This point is where I came in. As ever, I had not considered researching Clary Sage, but on that brightly moonlit night before the lunar eclipse a would-be healer asked a question in a Facebook soapmaking forum about recipes to help a friend who was struggling to get pregnant because she had PCOS, and the asker had read that Clary Sage would be a good oil to choose to boost fertility.

We can't argue with the logic of the thoughts can we?

But then at 4.30am a random thought entered my mind and refused to let me sleep...

But PCOS has an oestrogen dominant environment

And not matter how hard I have wracked my brains I cannot recall how I even *knew* that, but let's go over why Clary Sage would not be the best choice for helping fertility when a woman has PCOS.

What is PCOS?

Around about 5% of the women have PCOS making it a fairly common disease. About 20% of the general population have polycystic ovaries, but it is not yet understood whether this is a reliable indicator of whether PCOS will manifest.

So far, there is little understanding of why it happens, although it is believed to be intricately linked with the mechanisms controlling insulin.

Insulin's job is to control blood sugar and if the body becomes insulin resistant then cells are not longer able to process it and it remains and accumulates in the blood stream. This leads to problems such as obesity, diabetes and a disturbed menstrual cycle which in turn makes fertility very difficult.

Irregular Periods

Often indicators of PCOS can be seen very early on in puberty when there are irregular and very heavy periods. Now this should point to a misfire in the hormones triggering ovulation, but orthodox treatment for these painful periods is the contraceptive pill which helps to bring "the cycle" into line. The pill does help the pain and because it is an artificial cycle, the problem is masked and may not become apparent until the women comes off contraceptive, symptoms reappear and we now discover she will have trouble conceiving. In other words, treating her symptoms allopathically may have *seemed* to have made her better, but actually the problem never went away (although it became less problematic day to day) and when the mask is taken off the root cause looks the same.

Androgenic Symptoms

Often women with PCOS will have higher levels of a group of hormones called androgens. The best recognised of this set of chemicals is testosterone which means often there will be an excess of body or facial hair and some darkening of the pigmentation in the arm pit. Sometimes there will be a receding hair line or hair thinning too.

Obesity

This is a no win situation because weight gain will affect the insulin causing weight gain , which in turn affects the follicles and then also it is really hard to lose the weight because of it. About 40% of women with PCOS are overweight. The good news is that a weight reduction of just 5% can begin to improve ovarian function.

Diagnosing PCOS is a several pronged approach the doctor's help will be vital here, to deciding which essential oils to choose for treatment and whether Clary Sage would be the correct choice.

Firstly the doc will appraise the presenting symptoms, the menstrual history, weight and hair situation, for example. Then he will proceed to blood tests which are our best friend.

He will test for androgens and SHBG, (sex hormone binding globulin – shows excess testosterone in women). Next he will check the various hormones connected to ovulation so FSH, LH and oestrogen. The classic profile would look like:

- High LH
- Low Oestrogen

Finally at day 21, he will take another test to see if ovulation has taken place.

Now, that looks in direct opposition to what I previously said, doesn't it? I said oestrogen dominant environment, but we see low oestrogen production in the ovaries...

This is because another set of oestrogen comes from another source, and as yet it is not clear where. Some sources suggest it might be the fat cells themselves creating the oestrogen. It could be the cysts, or the oestrogen may *cause* the cysts. Other possible theories are that the oestrogen dominance mat come from an external factor: the environment, as well as lifestyle or genetics.

Of particular interest are *xenoestrogens, manmade chemicals that mimic oestrogen and disr*upt our internal ecology. These can lay dormant in the fat cells for decades. Pesticides sprayed onto crops and growth hormones given to livestock and poultry are also thought to be possible culprits.

In most women then, one would expect to see PCOS causing an oestrogen dominant environment (unless other case history details make you suspect deficiency,) Clary Sage would be the wrong treatment to choose for menstrual/ fertility issues. To repeat, what I mentioned earlier, I would opt for Vitex Agnus Castus, also known as chasteberry instead, to boost progesterone. Clearly ylang ylang, re and geranium all help in various mechanisms to *balance* the hormones too.

Perimenopause

You can pretty much repeat what I wrote above. Even though oestrogen is receding, there is a dearth of progesterone because there is no longer a corpus luteum to create the hormone. Again then, we go vitex, ylang, rose, geranium

Menopause

Menstruation is regulated and eased by Clary Sage and her anti spasmodic actions. Again, we must ask ourselves is it this oestrogenic quality that pacifies and eases the blood flow...? As yet, we cannot say *scientifically* that it is! We can however attribute it to the antispasmodic effects of the esters.

Isn't science confusing?!!

I recently wrote a piece about the psychological aspects of menopause for National Association of Holistic Aromatherapists and the research quite set my brain into a spin.

We know menopause benefits from Clary Sage's uplifting and antidepressant quality. But, I wondered, does this come from some hormonal effect or do more ancient clues hold the key? Many psychological studies are starting to uncover a pattern of connections about how we feel about going through menopause, and the actual symptoms we experience. There are many studies comparing different cultures and their attitudes towards the end of fertility and the effects that women from that culture complain of. As an English woman, I confess to being quite afraid of getting old. My grandmother had breast cancer and so I have worried for many years that I would not be able to have HRT and would become "old" very quickly if I had a hysterectomy. Reading these studies made me question what being "old" translated to me. I worried about my skin drying up, weight gain, mood swings, hot flushes and night sweats, brittle bones and a loss of my femininity.

I was shocked to find only night sweats and hot flushes actually had a physiological link with the hormonal changes that happen through menopause. Whilst all of the other symptoms connected with our perceptions of menopause are very real complaints, they come from some other unknown source. What's more, a woman from a different country might complain of a completely different menopausal experience entirely. Mayan women and women from parts of rural Greece for instance, describe no menopausal symptoms at all, except for a cessation of bleeding.

How about that for strange? It certainly gave me pause!

It seems Mayan women in particular, get married very young, about the age of twelve. They go on to have many, many children and hardly have any periods at all. They believe that the menopause is simply that they have used up all their blood in childbirth and when it ends, they do not mourn the loss of fertility, because they have many children. They then go onto a far freer way of life. They can go to church and see their friends, free of "blooding" and also I suspect young children too. When asked about how their husband's felt about the end of their fertility, they very pragmatically asked "what's it got to do with them? They didn't have to endure the blooding, did they?" Theirs, too, I feel is a culture of reverence for the elderly, where the crone holds a place of great esteem. In England, I am ashamed to say that is not so.

Now moon medicine is about that which is held in shadow. Whilst some would say our unconscious mind, I would prefer to describe it as those thoughts that come unconsciously, perhaps through conditioning. The moon medicine of Clary Sage challenges these perceptions and peels back the layers of our symptoms to the undercurrents of our childhood and values that could be causing our anxiety and stress responses.

Pregnancy

The big one. I was always taught you do not use Clary Sage until 37 weeks, and that it will bring on labour. By the same token, I always say no essential oils *at all* in the first 16 weks of pregnancy

To quote from the NAHA:

Jane Buckle comments "the use of essential oils in pregnancy is a contentious subject, especially during the vital first 3-month period. It is extremely unlikely that a nightly bath containing a few drops of essential oils will cause any problems for the unborn child" and later states "there are no records of abnormal fetuses or aborted fetuses due to the 'normal' use of essential oils, either by inhalation or topical application."

According to Wildwood, "A common myth in aromatherapy is that massage oils containing essential oils such as Clary Sage, rose or even

rosemary can cause a miscarriage and hence should be avoided throughout
pregnancy. Authors such as Ron Guba, Kurt Schnaubelt, and Chrissie
Wildwood have all pointed out that there have been 'no recorded cases of
miscarriage or birth defect resulting from aromatherapy massage using
therapeutic applications of any essential oil."

Personally, I stick to the 37 week guideline, but I have to say I see no evidence of it bringing on early labour. I have used it in three of my own pregnancies and also on some friends. Labour has followed fairly quickly behind, but then at 37 weeks...it should! That said, everything I have seen shows that contractions are more efficient are less painful, and labour is shorter when it is used. Is that because of the oestrogen, or because it calms the mother so panic cannot slow contractions? Dunno. Don't care. It works. That's what counts.

You might also find it interesting to read the foundation study of a massive trial of aromatherapy in a maternity ward. http://www.scirp.org/journal/PaperDownload.aspx?paperID=43420

Gabriel Mojay describes the actions thus: "In terms of Oriental medicine, Clary Sage oil both strengthens Qi-energy that is depleted, and relaxes and circulates Qi-energy that is "stuck". Hence it is both an effective general tonic and a major antispasmodic. As such then, we can imagine the better blood flow from its vasodilatory action. We might think of constipation, colic, varicose veins, indigestion or phlegm. Where the internal functions become sluggish and lazy, then Clary Sage is useful.

Breast Milk

I have to tell you a lovely story. Whilst I have been writing this book, I had an SOS from French aromatherapist Mischa Ichikawa. She had a dear friend staying with her with a new baby who was very restless. She asked what I used for encouraging breast milk production and I explained that even though these impressive mammaries look like they should lactate gold top, I had been unable to successfully feed any of my children for very long, but that personally I would have chosen celery seed and dill. She said she had read Clary Sage, and what did I think of that? Makes sense, I thought and so we went with it.

Here's a paste of my thoughts:

I wouldn't put it on the breasts per se. Use it in her bath perhaps? The oils will absorb into the blood stream, or perhaps she could use some warm compresses?

Compresses on her boobs obviously!

1 drop is enough whatever the carrier I think, in case baby does not like the taste.

Another thing I learned that was useful...The very first smell baby recognises is colostrum. Apparently it smells the same as amniotic fluid...although how they know that I have no idea but...when baby goes quiet when he is being held and then cries when he is put in his cot, it is because he can no longer smell the colostrums.

Now clearly hers has gone, but it might be worth expressing some milk onto his sheets to nuzzle up to.

Perhaps give mum a shoulder or back massage with the oils to calm her. Rose as well... just so her stress drops because then his will too. Babies' cortisol mimics mums.

Mischa's reply, 2 days later:

Well we decided on one drop Clary Sage in a tbspn about in my palm and massaged down her spine (like that, far enough from baby & read it's a good place to apply) and it worked!! She had lots more milk that night, so I gave her the bottle & her hubby will do it for her. Powerful stuff!!

Respiratory

Potentially I have not touched on respiratory actions anywhere near as much as I should. These are useful on several levels. The antispasmodic action releases the grip of asthma. It is gently sedative to sore throats and relieves the coughing. Salvatore Battaglia tells us "Clary Sage is recommended for treating asthma as it relaxes spasms in the bronchial tube and helps reduce anxiety and emotional tension often associated with asthma sufferers. Mojay's comments about energizing qi help us to comprehend that we can use Clary Sage and expect phlegm to start to move. The energy release opens the chest and eases feelings of constriction.

If we think back to the oestrogen note though, you may recall that oestrogen helps nitric oxide to dilate the blood vessels in the cells walls. This nitric oxide forms a fundamental part of my Bronchitis book, as is complicated but suffice it to say when oestrogen opens the membranes the gas exchange makes breathing easier.

Aphrodisiac

Would I put this top of the list of the down and dirties…no, probably not. Ylang ylang, tuberose and vetiver would be my go to's but…

I think if a long term relationship has been going through the mill and it needs a moment where bickering is replaced by a "Ooo yes, I kinda remember what I saw in you" moment, then Clary Sage is good.

The same applies for reigniting the fire that menopause has dampened. Clary Sage moistens in a far more exciting way.

If memories and traumas are preventing you from relaxing into the moment, then again, yes give Clary Sage a try. Often good aromatherapy is very much suck it and see…just like good sex, really! There are no rules, only great opportunities.

Skin Care

It's not really an oil that would immediately spring to mind for skin care, but it does have its uses. It is astringent and it is very gentle. Use it to cut through grease and grime, but also to hydrate the skin. Using Clary Sage over time will bring a beautiful dewy effect to the skin.

Musical Note

A major or F sharp minor (Both have 3 sharps in the key signature and funnily enough sound very different when they are played!)

We'll start with F sharp minor and its angry aggressive tone.

So, there are no prizes for guessing what the first song is going to be. Written in F#, it opens with the words...

"I hate the world today"

Bitch – Meredith Books

https://www.youtube.com/watch?v=rhfiiGGy7Ls

Meredith tells her lover...

Rest assured that

When I start to make you nervous

And I'm going to extremes

Tomorrow I will change

And today won't mean a thing

Chuckle...this should be my anthem. My poor husband!

Sing it ladies. Get that Clary Sage prescription rammed into your brain.

Pink- So What?

https://www.youtube.com/watch?v=FJfFZqTlWrQ

The fabulous Pink's feeling the Clary Sage note in her song "So what?" The moon kicks every last bit of care in mercury's relationship. Uh-uh... you know what's coming don't you?

I don't want you tonight,

You weren't there,

I'm gonna show you tonight,

I'm alright,

I'm just fine,

And you're a tool,

So, so what,

I am a rock star,

I got my rock moves,

And I don't want you tonight!

Yep:

Na na na na na na na I wanna start a fight,

Prayer of the Refugee

https://www.youtube.com/watch?v=0TC_-cU2FiU

Next, we have pre-linalool aggression of refugees. The terrifying anger of those ripped from their homes to a supposedly better place, only to be greeted by a different hostility. Moon's medicine wants to know what the bloody hell happened?

Warm yourself by the fire, son,

And the morning will come soon.

I'll tell you stories of a better time,

In a place that we once knew.

Before we packed our bags

And left all this behind us in the dust,

We had a place that we could call home,

And a life no one could touch.

And perhaps the drunken rage as someone tries to soothe him and remove him from a club. Wherever he is, he ain't happy!

Don't hold me up now,

I can stand my own ground,

I don't need your help now,

You will let me down, down, down!

Prayer of the refugee is terrifying in its fury. Solemn storytelling, explosive rage, pride and embarrassment.

Land of Confusion

https://www.youtube.com/watch?v=1pkVLqSaahk

Genesis uses the same key that Clary Sage resonates in to create their song Land of Confusion. And as we think of that horrible research into Alzheimer's I am going to use their words to beg you to use this research to ease some of the myriad pains you see manifest around you. The entire song makes me angry thinking about all the silly arguments going on about how we should and shouldn't use aromatherapy. It's the healing that counts! Get off facebook, out of the argumentative point scoring forums and go massage someone. It could make all the difference in the world.

There's too many men

Too many people

Making too many problems

And not much love to go round

Can't you see

This is a land of confusion.

This is the world we live in

And these are the hands we're given

Use them and let's start trying

To make it a place worth living in

Stone Sour – Looking Through the Glass

https://www.youtube.com/watch?v=vBfb3IFhu9o

When the moon clouds the mercury vibration, we want to go home and lick our wounds. We alienate those around us and feel separated from the reality everyone else can see.

Stone Sour captures this beautifully in their enigmatic ballad.

No-one ever tells you that forever feels like home, sitting all alone, sitting all alone inside your head.

The lines *"How do you feel? That is the question But I forget, you don't expect an easy answer* seem like they could only have been written by a hormonal gal!

Behind Blue Eyes – Limp Biscuit

https://www.youtube.com/watch?v=fEGI9NbH-mkthe

Please don't get angry at me for not choosing The Who's version. You don't get Fred Durst's torso in that one!

No one knows what it's like

To be the bad man

To be the sad man

Behind blue eyes

And no one knows

What it's like to be hated

To be fated to telling only lies

Hormones perhaps?

I Feel It in My Bones – The Killers

https://www.youtube.com/watch?v=ECHv5KV4ZuM

You might say history's strangest Christmas song is about Santa Claus...looks more like osteoporosis and menopause to me!

Nights have been restless, pillows and sheets

Bet you got it all figured out

I sweat like a snowman out in the sun

Dreaming that there ain't nowhere to run to, baby

Nowhere to hide

And I feel it in my bones

And I feel it in my bones

Enough of the anger, then. Let's go into the key of A major.

Let's have something beautiful now. None lovelier than **The Way We Were – Barbara Streisand.**

https://www.youtube.com/watch?v=GNEcQS4tXgQ

Mem'ries,

Light the corners of my mind

Misty water-colored memories

Of the way we were

Scattered pictures,

Of the smiles we left behind

Smiles we gave to one another

For the way we were

And so finally, what better place to end than the song about aging, memories and fading loveliness cursed by the moonlight.

Memory- Elaine Paige

https://www.youtube.com/watch?v=4-L6rEm0rnY

Midnight

Not a sound from the pavement

Has the moon lost her memory?

She is smiling alone

In the lamplight, the withered leaves collect at my feet

And the wind begins to moan

Memory

All alone in the moonlight

I can smile at the old days

I was beautiful then

I remember the time I knew what happiness was

Let the memory live again

Every streetlamp seems to beat a fatalistic warning

Someone mutters, and a streetlamp gutters,

And soon it will be morning.

Daylight

I must wait for the sunrise

I must think of a new life

And I mustn't give in.

When the dawn comes, tonight will be a memory too

And a new day will begin

Burnt out ends of smokey days

The stale cold smell of morning

The streetlamp dies, another night is over

Another day is dawning...

Touch me!

It's so easy to leave me

All alone with the memory

Of my days in the sun...

If you touch me, you'll understand what happiness is

Look, a new day

Has begun

Recipes

Just a quick reminder of our prevailing issues with this oil to save me from writing the same contraindications over and over....

My recommendation is not to use before 37 weeks of pregnancy. Do not drink alcohol or take mind altering drugs with Clary Sage. That's not a nice trip and it will provoke a headache. Using too much CS also causes a headache so we keep dosage slow.

Oh...and if you use it right...It provoketh the venery! Make sure you have got your good knickers on!

Clary Sage for Period Pains

As the clinical trials show, there is no specific way to achieve this reduction in pain. Whether you use it just on period days, or choose to treat the body in a cycle, both should be affective. From a personal point of view, it makes sense to treat through the month and then ramp it up on the bad days.

In the same way, most effective is going to be massaging onto the abdomen, but again, I would also rub into the lower back to work on receptors that give us lower back pain when the demon days descend.

Start today!

50ml (2 fl oz) Rosehip Carrier

Clary Sage x 2

Rose x 1

Fennel x 1

Here I have used fennel, which is another oil believed to have slightly oestrogenic effects, but is also very good to tackle the bloating and water retention we expect later in the month. Let's get in early!

Use on days 1 – 5 of cycle (day on being first day of period)

50ml (2 fl oz) Rosehip Carrier

Clary Sage x 2

Rose x 1

Lavender x 2

Camomile Roman x 2

Then revert to blend 1 again.

Clary Sage for Labour

Start using after week 37.

50ml (2 fl oz) Evening Primrose Oil

Rose x 2

Clary Sage x 4

Frankincense x 2

I chose Evening Primrose because this too, is full of prostaglandins that kick of labour. Possibly TMI but I used this with Dex's pregnancy as an internal massage on the perineum too, to stop tearing!

Clary Sage in Established Labour

When things are definitely under way and mum is comfortably ensconced in hospital or home in readiness for the big event, we can strengthen the contractions, ease the pain and make for happier mum and baby.

Take the existing blend and add some more oils in to make it into

50ml (2 fl oz) Evening Primrose Oil

Rose x 2

Clary Sage x 8

Frankincense x 2

Jasmine x 1

Myrrh x 1

Lavender x 5

Hello little baby…you'll be showing your face in no time.

Aromatherapy for Peri-menopausal Symptoms

Anxiety and Depression

50ml (2oz) blank moisturizer or carrier oil

Vitex Agnus Castus x 2

Rose x 1

Geranium x 1

Of course, there is no need to always be focussing on hormones and so we could just go sedative or uplifting too.

Sedative

50g (2 oz) Sea salt

Vetiver x 1

Geranium x 1

Mandarin x 1

(Note we have deliberately stayed away from Clary Sage because of the low levels of progesterone)

Sensuality

50ml (2 fl oz) Rosehip Carrier

Rose x 1

Sandalwood x 1

Ylang ylang x 1

This is a nice one because the heady fragrance of ylang ylang is sensuous, but of course it is a hormonal balancer too.

Clary Sage for Menopause

Hot Flushes

Clearly we need the most cooling help we can get here, and peppermint ranks as that it my mind. The problem is, though, if we splash that on with gusto that the flushes require…we are going to be awake all night, so I think going for a homeopathic dose makes the most sense. So, we are making just $1/15^{th}$ of a drop.

Count out 14 drops of carrier oil, I use sunflower oil because it is cheap. Add one drop of peppermint.

Bottle it.

Use one drop of the mix.

Peppermint x 1/15th drop

Clary Sage x 2

Spikenard x 1

Rose x 1

Cooling Spritz

50ml (2 fl oz) Rose hydrolat

25ml (2 fl oz) Clary Sage hydrolat

25ml (2 fl oz) spikenard hydrolat

Decant into a spray bottle

Night Sweats

We are going on the same pretext as the above, but this is written from the viewpoint of someone who has to go to bed toastie- warm!

So rather than cooling, we are aiming to reduce the actual fluid loss from the sweating, if that makes sense. Spikenard is cooling, but ginger is a specific for any condition where the body is struggling to cope with moisture. Patchouli reduces sweating. Again, I am going homeopathic with the ginger otherwise I think we would feel volcanic!

Count out 14 drops of carrier oil, I use sunflower oil because it is cheap. Add one drop of ginger.

Bottle it.

Use one drop of the mix.

Night Sweat Bath Salts

100g Sea Salt

Clary Sage x 2

Spikenard x 3

Ginger x 1/15th drop

Patchouli x 2

Clary Sage for Insomnia

This blend is relaxing but it relies on actions of the Central Nervous System to try to reset the body clock over time. Clearly, you could just as easily diffuse this, find a handsome and willing bloke to massage you or whack these oils in the bath. Rub onto the neck and insides of the wrist 1/2 hour before bed time

50ml (2 fl oz) blank lotion

Lavender x 2

Clary Sage x 1

Marjoram x 1

Clary Sage for Anxiety

Because the energy of anxiety is very yin, up in the air, floaty and slightly out of your brain, I use yang oils to drag the patient down and anchor the energy down.

I think I'll go evaporator oils here.

Vetiver grounds and calms, sweet basil instils confidence to stand up and face what is worrying you.

Clary Sage x 1

Sweet Basil x1

Vetiver x 1

Or we could go neroli for liquid tranquiliser and base note benzoin to stick the feet down on terra firma.

Clary Sage x 1

Neroli   x 1

Benzoin x 1

I *can* Face the Day Shower Gel
330ml shower Gel

Clary Sage x 4

Basil x 2

Grapefruit x 2

Clary Sage for Clear Thinking
We might be talking about our poor dementia patients, panicked students or better decision making in depression.

How about a lovely refreshing flannel to lift the spirits and try to touch some old memories?

Fill a bowl with hand hot water. Add:

1 x Clary Sage

1 x Rose

1 x Melissa

Perhaps add a drop of lavender on days when they are very stressed. Soak the flannel, squeeze out and gently place on the face for a compassionate face wash.

Clary Sage Revision Help

My mum wrote in her book *The Garden of Eden* (Jill Bruce) "An oil to help with conversations and mathematics" and that made me smile because remember Mercury is the father of Maths. My son is a mathematician, and there is something very clear sighted about the revelations an equation uncovers. He is very certain when he has got something right and becomes very calm when a problem is solved. Yes, I can see how CS would be like maths.

We can help their concentration, their insights and their nerves here. How about making some aromatherapy pencils?

Use unvarnished pencils, and paint over the wood. Alternatively, use in a diffuser, or maybe in a shower gel to boost them in the morning before school.

Rosemary x 1

Clary Sage x 1

Vetiver x 1

Clary Sage For Meditation

Whilst it is not quite magic mushrooms, Clary Sage is most definitely a plant with connections to the inner realm. Given people's assertions that Clary Sage is euphoric perhaps we should be talking about Lucy in the Sky with Diamonds but...

It is a brilliant oil to use in meditation when you have a decision to make which is clouded by emotion.

It is a great oil to use if you are struggling to get a creative project off the ground and you are not quite sure where to take it next. Clary Sage helps you to make your ideas manifest.

As a moon baby, I use my evaporator out in the garden between the plants under the moonlight...but hey. Each to their own. Quietness is all we require.

Clary Sage x 1

Monarda x 1

Nutmeg x 1

Clary Sage for Depression

I have written several blend here because I think the nature of depression isto think "nothing is going to work" and to have a low adherence to using a blend. Conversely, studies show we need to use the oils over time to see a marked effect, so change and change about. Use in diffusers, baths, massage oils, there are no rules. The only restriction you have is your own imagination.

Blend 1

Rose x 1

Clary Sage x 1

Geranium x 1

Blend 2

Bergamot x 1

Clary Sage x 1

Myrrh x 1

Blend 3

Mandarin x 1

Clary Sage x 1

Benzoin x 1

Blend 4

Cypress X 1

Clary Sage x1

Sandalwood x 1

Blend 5

Lemon x 1

Clary Sage x 1

Vetiver x 1

Blend 6

This is a lovely fresh green blend that I have fallen in love with! I have made it into an Eau De Toilette. It is like spring happiness.

Lemon verbena x 1

Clary Sage x 1

Gingergrass x 1

(See my 75 Christmas Gift Ideas book to learn how to make perfume)

Clary Sage for Obsessive Compulsive Disorder

50ml (2 fl oz) Moisturiser

Clary Sage x 2

Vetiver x 1

Valerian x 1

For the first fortnight, use five times a day, then drop down to morning and night. Either rub onto the back of the neck or on the insides of the wrists.

Clary Sage for Sensuality

Bath Salts

100g (4 oz) Sea salts

Rose x 1

Clary Sage x1

Vetiver x 1

Sensual Massage Oil

50ml (2 fl oz) Massage oil

Tuberose x 1

Clary Sage x 1

Sandalwood x 1

Clary Sage from Muscular Aches and Pains

50ml (2 fl oz) Blank Ointment

Clary Sage x 2

Lavender x 4

Juniper x 2

It makes sense too, to extend this blend to osteoarthritis because the oils will deal with the uric acid but Clary Sage may also help the oestrogenic aspect.

Clary Sage for The Respiratory System

Clary Sage is a very useful oil to use for problems such as asthma because of its antispasmodic effects. It relaxes the bronchial tubes and of course it helps reduce the anxiety that accompanies the disease and its attacks.

During an attack, if you can calm the patient to take a couple of gasps of the fumes from the bottle, this is useful. The same applies for a tablespoon of the hydrolat. Breathing oils will also calm the panic.

Asthma Massage Oil

40ml (1 ½ fl oz) Tamanu oil

10ml (½ fl oz Sea Buckthorn oil)

Clary Sage x 1

Frankincense x 1

Niaouli x 1

Massage onto the chest and back twice a day.

Bronchitis Treatment

Because as Mojay states, Clary Sage helps stasis, this is a good oil to attack not only the breathing but the mucous build-up of congestion.

Use as an inhalation

Put drops into hot water, with a towel over your head. Try to breathe through your mouth.

Clary Sage x 1

Myrrh x 1

Lemon x 1

Clearly you can use this as a cream or massage oil too.

Coughs

Heat a mug of apple juice. Add:

Clary Sage x 1

Myrtle x 1

Camomile x 1

To a ½ tsp of honey to dissolve the oils.

Stir in and drink.

There are no vitamins in essential oils, but the apple juice is packed full of nutrients.

Clary Sage for Clear Eyes

Make cold compresses with rosewater and a drop of Clary Sage to rinse out foreign bodies, and to ease the soreness of conjunctivitis.

Clary Sage for Cleaning Wounds

Use a cold compress with the following

Clary Sage x 3

Tea Tree x 2

Lavender x 1

Clary Sage Drawing Ointment

Alternating hot and cold compresses makes a kind of suction effect, drawing toxins and foreign bodies to the surface. You could use the oils to draw out in that way too, using a hot compress for five minutes, then a cold one for five, repeat for three cycles.

1 tbs Kaolin powder

Clary Sage x 1

Juniper x 1

Cypress x 2

Mix to a stiff paste with a couple of drops of water. Place over the boil / abscess and cover with a dry dressing. Leave over night.

Clary Sage for Constipation

50ml (2 fl oz) Sunflower oil

Coriander x 2

Clary Sage x 1

Ginger x 1

Massage around the belly button in a clockwise direction. Use twice a day to ease discomfort and tone the digestive system.

Clary Sage for Varicose Veins

25ml (1 fl oz) Aqueous cream

25ml (1 fl oz) water

Geranium x 1

Clary Sage x 1

Cypress x 1

Mix well. Stroke into the legs, twice a day.

Clary Sage for Restless Legs

1tbs Epsom salts

Clary Sage x 1

Valerian x 1

Lavender x 1

In the bath at the end of the day. Peaceful sleep ensured.

Hydrating Moisturiser for Greasy skin

50ml (2 fl oz) Blank moisturiser

Clary Sage x 1

Lavender x 1

Ylang Ylang x 1

Dewy Skin Tonic

50ml Clary Sage hydrolat

Clary Sage x 1

Rose x 1

Geranium x 1

Shampoo For Greasy Hair and Dandruff

Add to your 330ml bottle of usual shampoo

Clary Sage x 4

Petitgrain x 6

Patchouli x 6

Deep Cleansing Masque for all skin types

1 tbs Green Clay

1 tsp Borage Carrier Oil

Clary Sage x 1

Carrot x 1

Myrrh x 1

Cypress x 2

Leave on the skin for 5 minutes then rinse off with warm water. Follow with toner and moisturiser.

Conclusion

It's quite hard, isn't it, not having scientific evidence to fall back on? This book has felt like a lesson in patience, although I don't know why, because there was very little clinical evidence available when I trained.

Endocrinology was always my favourite part of my Anatomy and Physiology course, and every day that passion deepens. I think if I had my time over again, I would have wanted to be a psychiatrist. I hope that perhaps some of my notes about the oil might help some of the tortured souls being in nurtured in institutions because their sanity eloped with an errant hormone never to be seen again. To think Clary Sage might be able to help these people feels like the most exquisite pain to me.

On the most mundane levels, though, we can help alleviate the period pains that take over people's lives. We can more confidently try to help people who want to become pregnant and probably most important of all we can better the lives of women locked in a hell created by menopause. If our medicine only helps to relieve their anxiety and lift their depression then frankly, my work here is done.

I have an enormous number of "thank you"s with this book. Firstly and most importantly my friend Fay who patiently waited for a child to appear when Clary Sage, frankly ,did not speed up labour very much at all. It is thanks to Fay and her daily nagging that I even began to write these books. Her friendship and belief in me have genuinely changed my life.

Thank you too to Annelise Manchanda Piers and the ladies and gentlemen of the Soapmaking With Natural Ingredients forum on facebook for asking the initial question about Clary Sage and fertility.

To Gergely Hollodi and the staff at Aromatika.hu for the idea to write about CS. To Robert Tisserand for not laughing out loud at my madness over Clary Sage Seed oil. To Misha Ichikawa and her lovely breast milk research and to the breastfeeding mum, Bilitis Trumeau, for allowing me to tell her tale.

The book is dedicated to Zuzana and her son. She is a translator who, without fail, sends me a reply to my newsletters and is always the first person to tell me what she thinks of my books. She is just one of hundreds of voices in the wilderness who make writing these books worthwhile for me. Your feedback and conversation is like oxygen to my work. When it goes quiet out there it becomes very hard to know there is a purpose to what I am doing. I am deeply grateful to all of you for your love and support. So please, don't forget to comment and leave reviews and even if you are really impressed with my ideas pop over to Real Aromatherapy Reviews on facebook and say what you think there. All of these help me to sell books which in turn mean I can afford to keep up the work!

As ever, be gentle on yourselves. Experiment with the oil and please let me know how you get on.

Don't forget

Review and buy…

Bye!

Liz

PS. Just for the record, these last words were written and the book finally uploaded to the publishing software on Nov 25th. Tonight is the full moon.... Let's hope She is pleased.

About the Author

Elizabeth Ashley qualified as an aromatherapist in 1993, and then passed her Advanced Aromatherapy Diploma in 1994. She has been practicing aromatherapy for almost 22 years.

In 1999, she fell into a whole new career in the aggressive commercial sector of recruitment consultancy. There she discovered her father's second hand car salesman genes had passed along and found she had quite a gift of the gab! More than that, she discovered she could sell...and then some.

In 2008, Elizabeth fell ill during pregnancy with a blood clot in her lungs. The pulmonary embolism prevented her from working and she started to write. Very quickly she gained her first contract as a ghost writer...a recipe book for cheese cakes!

In 2010 she was published professionally for her work on Galbanum - (Ferula Galbaniflua) oil in the Aromatherapy Thymes, journal of the International Federation of Aromatherapists, and on TubeRose - (Rosa damascena) oil by the New Zealand Register of Holistic Therapist.

In 2011 she was seconded on a consultative basis to Walsall Independent Treatment Centre, designed to be a rainbow bridge between traditional and complementary medicines. There she became aware of the rumblings of change in healthcare. Her book Sales Strategies for Gentle Souls explains the connotations of this.

Many of her books are aimed at helping qualified aromatherapists to expand their healing repertoire and build their businesses. She also writes for people who have an interest in essential oils and want to learn how to heal. Her in depth essential oil profiles chart the healing properties of plants from the most arcane depths of historic folklore up to the scientific lab trials of today.

In 2014 she ranks in the top 50 contract writers on the freelancer marketplace Elance.com. She is the ghost writer of seven number one Amazon best sellers in the natural healing category. She lives in Shropshire with her husband and youngest son, kept company by their cat, the budgie and many shoals of tropical fish! Her elder son and daughter attend University and make her prouder than anything ever could.

Elizabeth Ashley is possibly one of the most published aromatherapy writers you have never heard of! By 2015, all of that will have changed. Elizabeth Ashley is The Secret Healer.

Other Books by the Author

Why not check out my reviews?

75 Quick and Easy Aromatherapy Christmas Gifts Ideas: Essential Oil Recipes For Handmade Personalised Gifts

50 Easy Essential Oil Recipes for Skin Care Products for Dry Skin - Make Your Own Anti-Aging Moisturizers & Night Creams

Professional Aromatherapy Skin Care Tips and Beauty Secrets

The Secret Healer Oils Profiles:

Some of the oils we have covered in this book will be familiar, but possibly not all. You may find some of the oils profiles deepen your knowledge and fascination for the art of aromatherapy.

Vetiver - (Vetiveria zizanoides): the Oil of Tranquillity

Monarda: A Native American Medicine

Holy Basil: An Ayurvedic Medicine

Rose - (Rosa damascena): Goddess Medicine; A Timeless Elixir

Sweet Basil - (Ocimum basilicum)– The Oil of Empowerment

The Secret Healing Manuals:

Book 1 - The Complete Guide to

Clinical Aromatherapy & Essential Oils for the Physical Body

Download for FREE

Book 2 Essential Oils for Mind Body Spirit

The Holistic Medicine of Clinical Aromatherapy

Book 3 The Essential Oil Liver Cleanse

The Professional Aromatherapist's Liver Detox

Book 4 The Professional Stress Solution

Essential Oils and Holistic Health Stress Management Techniques for The Professional Aromatherapist

Book 5 The Aromatherapy Eczema Treatment

Healing Eczema, Itchy Skin Rashes and Atopic Dermatitis with Essential Oils and Holistic Medicine

Book 6 The Aromatherapy Bronchitis Treatment

Support the Respiratory System with Essential Oils and Holistic Medicine for COPD, Emphysema, Acute and Chronic Bronchitis Symptoms

Sales Strategies for Gentle Souls; Targeted Sales Training for Professional Aromatherapists

Disclaimer

by SEQ Legal

(1)   Introduction

This disclaimer governs the use of this book. [By using this book, you accept this disclaimer in full. / We will ask you to agree to this disclaimer before you can access the book.]

(2)   Credit

This disclaimer was created using an SEQ Legal template.

(3)   No advice

The book contains information about aromatherapy and the use of essential oils.The information is not advice, and should not be treated as such.

[You must not rely on the information in the book as an alternative to qualified medical advice from a health professional. advice from an appropriately qualified professional. If you have any specific questions about any medical matter you should consult an appropriately qualified professional.]

[If you think you may be suffering from any medical condition you should seek immediate medical attention. You should never delay seeking medical advice, disregard medical advice, or discontinue medical treatment because of information in the book.]

(4)   No representations or warranties

To the maximum extent permitted by applicable law and subject to section 6 below, we exclude all representations, warranties, undertakings and guarantees relating to the book.

Without prejudice to the generality of the foregoing paragraph, we do not represent, warrant, undertake or guarantee:

that the information in the book is correct, accurate, complete or non-misleading;

that the use of the guidance in the book will lead to any particular outcome or result; or in particular, that by using the guidance in the book you will heal disease or work in any way as a cure for illness.

(5)   Limitations and exclusions of liability

The limitations and exclusions of liability set out in this section and elsewhere in this disclaimer: are subject to section 6 below; and govern all liabilities arising under the disclaimer or in relation to the book, including liabilities arising in contract, in tort (including negligence) and for breach of statutory duty.

We will not be liable to you in respect of any losses arising out of any event or events beyond our reasonable control.

We will not be liable to you in respect of any business losses, including without limitation loss of or damage to profits, income, revenue, use, production, anticipated savings, business, contracts, commercial opportunities or goodwill.

We will not be liable to you in respect of any loss or corruption of any data, database or software.

We will not be liable to you in respect of any special, indirect or consequential loss or damage.

(6)   Exceptions

Nothing in this disclaimer shall: limit or exclude our liability for death or personal injury resulting from negligence; limit or exclude our liability for fraud or fraudulent misrepresentation; limit any of our liabilities in any way that is not permitted under applicable law; or exclude any of our liabilities that may not be excluded under applicable law.

(7)   Severability

If a section of this disclaimer is determined by any court or other competent authority to be unlawful and/or unenforceable, the other sections of this disclaimer continue in effect.

If any unlawful and/or unenforceable section would be lawful or enforceable if part of it were deleted, that part will be deemed to be deleted, and the rest of the section will continue in effect.

(8)   Law and jurisdiction

This disclaimer will be governed by and construed in accordance with English law, and any disputes relating to this disclaimer will be subject to the exclusive jurisdiction of the courts of England and Wales.

(9)   Our details

In this disclaimer, "we" means (and "us" and "our" refer to) [Build Your Own Reality)] of [Sy8 1LQ].

Works Cited

Ashley, E. (2015). *Rose - Goddess Medicine; The Timeless Elixir of Ancient Egypt, Ayurveda, Chinese Medicine, Essential Oils and Modern Medicine* . Ludlow: Build Your Own Reality.

Barton, E. R. (2010, 12). *The G-protein-coupled estrogen receptor GPER in health and disease.* Retrieved 11 23, 2015, from Nature Revews - Endocrinology: http://www.nature.com/nrendo/journal/v7/n12/full/nrendo.2011.122 .html

Battaglia, S. (2002). *The Complete Guide To Aromatherapy* .

BBC.co.uk. (2003, 08 11). *Sex Hormone Controls Fear and Desire.* Retrieved 11 23, 2015, from BBC: http://news.bbc.co.uk/1/hi/uk/3142075.stm

Beck V1, U. E. (2003, 02). *Comparison of hormonal activity (estrogen, androgen and progestin) of standardized plant extracts for large scale use in hormone replacement therapy.* Retrieved 11 23, 2015, from Pubmed: http://www.ncbi.nlm.nih.gov/pubmed/12711012

Beck, T. (2012, 08). *Estrogen and Female Anxiety.* Retrieved 11 23, 2015, from Harvard Gazette:

http://news.harvard.edu/gazette/story/2012/08/estrogen-and-female-anxiety/

Beyene, Y. *From Menarche to Menopause: Reproductive Lives of Peasant Women in Two Cultures.* State University of New York Press.

Boots.com . (2015). *Women's health guide.* Retrieved 11 23, 2015, from http://www.webmd.boots.com/women/guide/oestrogen-womens-emotions

Boyles, S. (2003, 12 3). *Estrogen and The Stress Response.* Retrieved 11 23, 2015, from Web MD: http://www.webmd.com/depression/news/20031203/estrogen-is-involved-in-stress-response

Brace M1, M. E. (1997, 08). *Oestrogens and Psychological Wellbeing.* Retrieved 11 23, 2015, from Pubmed: http://www.ncbi.nlm.nih.gov/pubmed/9375984

Bull, J. L. (2000). *Aromatherapy and Subtle Energy Techniques: Compassionate Healing with Essential Oils.* North Atlantic Books,U.S.

Bussel, B. V. (1999, 08). *Moon.* Retrieved 11 23, 2015, from Busbi: http://busbi.home.xs4all.nl/moon.html

Buttler, R. (2009, 03 21). *Introduction to Archetypal Astrology: Sun, Moon, Mercury, Venus, and Mars.* Retrieved from Holotropic Breathwork: http://www.grof-holotropic-breathwork.net/group/archetypalholotropicastrology/forum/topics/introduction-to-archetypal

Changes in 5-hydroxy t rypt a mine and Cortis olPlasm a Leve ls in Menopausal Women Aft erInhalation of Clary Sage Oil†Kyung-Bok Lee, 1. C.-S. (2014, 07 05). *Changes in 5-hydroxy t rypt a mine and Cortis olPlasm a Leve ls in Menopausal Women Aft erInhalation of Clary Sage Oil.* Retrieved 11 23, 2015, from Readcube.com: http://www.readcube.com/articles/10.1002%2Fptr.5163?r3_referer=wol&tracking_action=preview_click&show_checkout=1&purchase_referrer=onlinelibrary.wiley.com&purchase_site_license=LICENSE_DENIED

Chavez C1, H. M. (2010, 03 19). *The effect of estrogen on dopamine and serotonin receptor and transporter levels in the brain: an autoradiography study.* Retrieved 11 23, 2015, from Pubmed: http://www.ncbi.nlm.nih.gov/pubmed/20079719

Clary Sage . (n.d.). Retrieved 11 23, 2015, from Inshanti: https://www.inshanti.com/t/more-info-clary-sage

Craig, M. (2013, 01). *Should psychiatrists be prescribing oestrogen therapy to their female patients?* Retrieved 11 23, 2015, from The British Journal of Psychiatry: http://bjp.rcpsych.org/content/202/1/9

Crow, D. (2006). *Clary Sage Peaceful Rejuvenation.* Retrieved 11 23, 2015, from Vedic Society: http://www.vedicsociety.org/clary-sage-peaceful-rejuvenation-a-245.html

Culpeppers Herbal Online. (n.d.). Retrieved from https://archive.org/details/cu31924001353279

David T. Zava, P. C. (1998, 03). *Estrogen and Progestin Bioactivity of Foods, Herbs, and Spices .* Retrieved 11 23, 2015, from Cancer Supportive Care: http://www.cancersupportivecare.com/estrogenherb.html

DE1., S. (2003, 04 25). *Menopause in highland Guatemala Mayan women.* Retrieved 11 23, 2015, from Pubmed: http://www.ncbi.nlm.nih.gov/pubmed/12697370

DeMarco, D. C. (n.d.). *Hormones forHealthy Menopause.* Retrieved 11 23, 2015, from Vitality Magazine: http://vitalitymagazine.com/article/hormones-for-healthy-menopause/

Dhillon, P. (2015). *How does Oestrogen Affect the Limbic Sytem in Females with Schizophrenia.* Retrieved 11 23, 2015, from Prezi: https://prezi.com/jkvxcapc8ndw/how-does-oestrogen-affect-the-limbic-system-in-females-with/

Dunkin J1, R. N.-S. (2005, 04 30). *Reproductive events modify the effects of estrogen replacement therapy on cognition in healthy postmenopausal women.* Retrieved 11 23, 2015, from Pubmed: http://www.ncbi.nlm.nih.gov/pubmed/15511602

Eden Botanicals. (n.d.). *Clary Sage Absolute.* Retrieved 11 23, 2015, from http://www.edenbotanicals.com/clary-sage-absolute.html

Emily Hayes, E. G. (2011, 11 10). *The Role of Oestrogen and Other Hormones in the Pathophysiology and Treatment of Schizophrenia.* Retrieved 11 23, 2015, from Schizophrenia Research and Treatment: http://www.hindawi.com/journals/schizort/2012/540273/

Epperson CN1, A. Z. (2013, 03). *Interactive effects of estrogen and serotonin on brain activation during working memory and affective processing in menopausal women.* Retrieved 11 23, 2015, from Pubmed: http://www.ncbi.nlm.nih.gov/pubmed/21820247

Estrogen . (n.d.). Retrieved 11 2015, 23, from Wikepedia: https://en.wikipedia.org/wiki/Estrogen

Farmer, D. J. (2014, 09 08). *Low Estrogen Common Casuses, Treatment and Symptoms.* Retrieved 11 23, 2015, from Nova Health Therapy: http://blog.novahealththerapy.com/hormones-and-your-health/low-estrogen-common-causes-symptoms-and-treatment-options

Fear Conditioning. (n.d.). Retrieved 11 23, 2015, from https://en.wikipedia.org/wiki/Fear_conditioning

Felson DT1, N. M. (1998, 05 10). *The effects of estrogen on osteoarthritis.* Retrieved 11 23, 2015, from Pubmed: http://www.ncbi.nlm.nih.gov/pubmed/9608332

Fink G1, S. B. (1996, 06 16). *Estrogen control of central neurotransmission: effect on mood, mental state, and memory.* Retrieved 11 23, 2015, from Pubmed: http://www.ncbi.nlm.nih.gov/pubmed/8818400

Gerard, J. (n.d.). *The English Herbal.* Retrieved from https://archive.org/details/cbarchive_121370_theherballorgeneralhis toryofpl1597

GJ1., t. H. (2010). *Effects of Estrogen on the Limbic System.* Retrieved 11 23, 2015, from Pubmed: http://www.ncbi.nlm.nih.gov/pubmed/20472146

Gören, G. T. (2007, 04 30). *Biological Activity of Diterpenoids Isolated from Anatolian.* Retrieved 11 19, 2015, from Reecords of Natural Products: http://www.acgpubs.org/RNP/2007/Volume%201/Issue%201/RNP07 _02.pdf

Gorney, C. (2010, 04 14). *The Estrogen Dilemma.* Retrieved 11 23, 2015, from New York Times Magazine: http://www.nytimes.com/2010/04/18/magazine/18estrogen- t.html?_r=0

Grahman, S. B. (2015, 11 09). *Menopause And Mood Disorders.* Retrieved 11 23, 2015, from Medscape: http://emedicine.medscape.com/article/295382-overview

Hitti, M. (2005, 06 08). *Estrogen Affects Obsessive Compulsive Disorder.* Retrieved 11 23, 2015, from Web MD: http://www.webmd.com/mental-health/news/20050608/estrogen-affects-obsessive-compulsive-disorder

Ho, S. P. (n.d.). *Attenuation of Fear Conditioning by antisense inhibition of brain corticotropin releasing factor-2 receptor.* Retrieved 11 23, 2015, from http://www.researchgate.net/publication/223351588_Attenuation_of_fear_conditioning_by_antisense_inhibition_of_brain_corticotropin_releasing_factor-2_receptor

Hodges, D. (2015, 10 23). *Clary Sage Oil.* Retrieved from Ayurvedic Oils.com: http://ayurvedicoils.com/tag/clary-sage-in-ayurveda

Hozzel, D. M. (2007, 04 29). *Clary Sage .* Retrieved 11 23, 2015, from Aromachat: http://www.aromachat.com/aromatherapy/clary-sage-salvia-sclarea-6/

http://www.ncbi.nlm.nih.gov/pubmed/10542441. (2011, 11). *Female Sex Homone as a Neuroprotectant.* Retrieved 11 23, 2015, from Pubmed: http://www.ncbi.nlm.nih.gov/pubmed/10542441

Hutchison JB1, B. C. (1994). *Gender-specific brain formation of oestrogen in behavioural development*. Retrieved 11 23, 2015, from Pubmed: http://www.ncbi.nlm.nih.gov/pubmed/7938352

Innes. (2013, 09 12). *Why Men Need Female Sex Hormones Too*. Retrieved 11 23, 2015, from Daily Mail: http://www.dailymail.co.uk/health/article-2418956/Why-men-need-womens-hormones-Oestrogen-vital-sex-drive-avoiding-obesity-say-doctors.html

Jayashri Kulkarni, 1. E. (2013, 07 01). *The Role of Estrogen in Treatment of Schizophrenia in Men*. Retrieved 11 23, 2015, from Pubmed: http://www.ncbi.nlm.nih.gov/pmc/articles/PMC3860106/

Jorge A Roman-Blas, 1. S.-B. (2009, 09 21). *Osteoarthritis associated with estrogen deficiency*. Retrieved 11 23, 2015, from Pubmed: http://www.ncbi.nlm.nih.gov/pmc/articles/PMC2787275/

K K Cover1, L. Y.-M. (2014, 08 05). *Mechanisms of estradiol in fear circuitry: implications for sex differences in psychopathology*. Retrieved 11 23, 2015, from Nature: http://www.nature.com/tp/journal/v4/n8/full/tp201467a.html

Laffayette Organics. (2015). *Clary Sage Oil* . Retrieved from Lafayette Organics: http://www.lafayetteorganics.com/essential-oils/clary-sage

Layton, J. (n.d.). *How Fear Works*. Retrieved 11 23, 2015, from How Stuff Works: Science : http://science.howstuffworks.com/life/inside-the-mind/emotions/fear7.htm

Levy, R. (2011, 07 11). *When Estrogen isn't the culpit*. Retrieved 11 23, 2015, from Harvard Gazette: http://news.harvard.edu/gazette/story/2011/07/when-estrogen-isn%E2%80%99t-the-culprit/

McCloskey, L. (2002). *Moon*. Retrieved 11 23, 2015, from Leigh McCloskey .com: http://www.leighmccloskey.com/Tarot/archetype_pages/moon.htm

McDermott, N. (2013, 07 10). *Why Women Cope Better With Stress Than Men*. Retrieved 11 23, 2015, from Daily Mail: http://www.dailymail.co.uk/health/article-2359132/Why-women-cope-better-stress-men-Oestrogen-helps-block-negative-effects-brain.html

MD Health. com. (2015). *Low Estrogen* . Retrieved 11 23, 2015, from MD Health: http://www.md-health.com/Low-Estrogen.html

Mojay, G. (1996). *Aromatherapy for Healing The Spirit*. Henry Holt and Company Inc.

Moon Conjunct Mercury. (n.d.). Retrieved 11 23, 2015, from Astro Matrix: http://astromatrix.org/Horoscopes/Planet-Aspects/Moon-Conjunct-Mercury

Moon Conjunct Mercury. (n.d.). Retrieved 11 23, 2015, from Dark Star Astrology: https://darkstarastrology.com/moon-conjunct-mercury/

Morgan MA1, P. D. (2001, 10). *Effects of Estrogen on Fear Related Behaviours in Mice.* Retrieved 11 23, 2015, from Pubmed: http://www.ncbi.nlm.nih.gov/pubmed/11716576

Northrup, C. (2015). *Estrogen Dominance.* Retrieved 11 23, 2015, from Dr Northrup MD: http://www.drnorthrup.com/estrogen-dominance/

Obsessive Behaviour Linked to Low Oestrogen Levels. (2008, 06 08). Retrieved 11 23, 2015, from New Scientist: https://www.newscientist.com/article/mg18625035-300-obsessive-behaviour-linked-to-low-oestrogen-levels/

Organic Facts. (n.d.). *Health Benefits of Clary Sage Essential Oil.* Retrieved 11 23, 2015, from https://www.organicfacts.net/health-benefits/essential-oils/health-benefits-of-clary-sage-essential-oil.html

Pederson, T. (2015). *Hormone Use In Menopause Lowers Depression and Anxiety.* Retrieved 11 23, 2015, from PsychCentral: http://psychcentral.com/news/2012/10/07/hormone-use-in-menopause-lowers-depression-anxiety-early/45683.html

Philipp Y Maximov, 1. T. (2013, 05 08). *The Discovery and Development of Selective Estrogen Receptor Modulators (SERMs) for*

Clinical Practice. Retrieved 11 23, 2015, from http://www.ncbi.nlm.nih.gov/pmc/articles/PMC3624793/

Pliny. (n.d.). *Natural History.* Retrieved from https://archive.org/stream/naturalhistory01plinuoft/naturalhistory01plinuoft_djvu.txt

Project Aware. (n.d.). *Progesterone Dominance.* Retrieved 11 23, 2015, from Project Aware: http://www.project-aware.org/index.shtml

Psych Education. org. (2014, 12). *Estrogen in Psychiatry.* Retrieved 11 23, 2015, from http://psycheducation.org/hormones-and-mood-introduction/basic-information-about-estrogen-in-psychiatry/

Quirk, G. J. (2002, 09 04). *Memory for Extinction of Conditioned Fear Is Long-lasting and Persists Following Spontaneous Recovery.* Retrieved 11 23, 2015, from Learning and Memory: http://learnmem.cshlp.org/content/9/6/402.full

Rashion, A. (1994). *Hormones in Havoc.* Retrieved 11 23, 2015, from Institute for Optimum Nutrition: http://www.ion.ac.uk/information/onarchives/hormoneshavoc3

RodneyYoung, R. a. (2013). *Essential Oil Safety: A Guide for Health Care Professionals.*

Salmon, W. (n.d.). *Botonalgia.* Retrieved from http://ia600709.us.archive.org/16/items/mobot31753003488134/mobot31753003488134.pdf

Sienkiewicz M1, G. A.-K. (2015, 02). *The effect of Clary Sage oil on staphylococci responsible for wound infections.* Retrieved 11 23, 2015, from Pubmed: http://www.ncbi.nlm.nih.gov/pubmed/25821423

Simone C. Mottaa, M. G. (2008, 05 08). *Dissecting the brain's fear system reveals the hypothalamus is critical for responding in subordinate conspecific intruders.* Retrieved 11 23, 2015, from Proceedings of The National Acedemy of Science of The United States of America: http://www.pnas.org/content/106/12/4870.full

Slary Sage Seed Oil. (2015). *CLARY SAGE SEED OIL* . Retrieved from Clary Seed.com: http://www.clarysageseedoil.com/

StillPoint. (n.d.). *Clary Sage Hydrosol.* Retrieved from http://www.stillpointaromatics.com/clary-sage-organic-hydrosol

Studd, P. J. (2010, 11 05). *The Treatment of Depression in Women By Oestrogens.* Retrieved 11 23, 2015, from www. studd.co.uk: http://www.studd.co.uk/dep_treatment.php

Sullivan, E. (2015). *The Sun and Moon* . Retrieved from Erin Sullivan.com: https://www.erinsullivan.com/articles/archetypal-psychological-astrology/109-sun-and-moon

Susan R. Davis, I. L. (2015, 04 23). *Menopause.* Retrieved 11 23, 2015, from Nature: http://www.nature.com/articles/nrdp20154

Susun Weed. (2000). *Clary Sage* . Retrieved 11 23, 2015, from http://www.susunweed.com/Article_ClarySage.htm

Synergy Essential Oils. (n.d.). *Clary Sage* . Retrieved 11 23, 2015, from http://www.synergyessentialoils.com/clary-sage

Temmen, M. (1999). *Clary Sage.* Retrieved 11 23, 2015, from Cheryls Herbs: http://cherylsherbs.com/Essential%20Oil%20Profiles/clarysage.htm

The Delicate Balance of PCOS and Estrogen Dominance. (2015). Retrieved 11 23, 2015, from PCOS Diva: http://pcosdiva.com/2014/09/delicate-balance-estrogen-dominance-pcos/

Theophastrus. (n.d.). *Enquiry Into Plants.* Retrieved from https://archive.org/stream/enquiryintoplant02theouoft/enquiryintoplant02theouoft_djvu.txt

Tisserand, R. (2010). *Is Clary Sage Estrogenic.* Retrieved from Robert Tisserand .com: http://roberttisserand.com/2010/04/is-clary-sage-oil-estrogenic/

Today. (2013, 09 13). *Oestrogen Plays a bit Role in Men's Bodies Too.* Retrieved 11 23, 2015, from http://www.todayonline.com/world/oestrogen-plays-big-role-mens-bodies-too

Towey, S. (n.d.). *Impact of Fear.* Retrieved 11 23, 2015, from University of Minnesota:

http://www.takingcharge.csh.umn.edu/enhance-your-wellbeing/security/facing-fear/impact-fear

Townsend EA1, M. L. (2011, 12). *Estrogen increases nitric-oxide production in human bronchial epithelium.* Retrieved 11 23, 2015, from Pubmed: http://www.ncbi.nlm.nih.gov/pubmed/21940647

Tree Frog Farm. (n.d.). *Clary Sage Flower Essence .* Retrieved 11 23, 2015, from http://www.treefrogfarm.com/store/flower-essences-tree-essences/clary-sage-flower-essence.html

W J Cutter, R. N. (2003). *Oestrogen, brain function, and neuropsychiatric disorders.* Retrieved 11 23, 2015, from Journal of Neurology, Neurosurgery and Psychiatry: http://jnnp.bmj.com/content/74/7/837.full

WebMD. (2015). *Estrogen and women's emotions .* Retrieved from Webmd: http://www.webmd.com/women/guide/estrogen-and-womens-emotions?page=2

What's Your Sign. (2005). *Mercury Symbol and Its Meanings .* Retrieved from Whats Your Sign : http://www.whats-your-sign.com/mercury-symbol.html

Williams, S. (2007, 12 26). *A Different Side To Estrogen.* Retrieved 11 23, 2015, from Science News: https://www.sciencenews.org/article/different-side-estrogen

Women's Health Concern. (n.d.). *Focus On Menopause*. Retrieved 11 23, 2015, from Women's Health Concern: http://www.womens-health-concern.org/help-and-advice/factsheets/focus-series/menopause/

Worwood, V. A. (2001). *Aromatherapy for the Beauty Therapist*. Cengage Learning Vocational.

Yoav Litvin*, G. C.-M. (2014, 05 21). *Estradiol regulates responsiveness of the dorsal premammillary nucleus of the hypothalamus and affects fear- and anxiety-like behaviors in female rats*. Retrieved 11 23, 2015, from European Journal of Neuroscience: http://onlinelibrary.wiley.com/doi/10.1111/ejn.12608/abstract

13808877R00088

Printed in Great Britain
by Amazon.co.uk, Ltd.,
Marston Gate.